Rob Labruyère

New outcome measures for subjects with incomplete spinal cord injury

Rob Labruyère

New outcome measures for subjects with incomplete spinal cord injury

Response time and adaptive walking

Südwestdeutscher Verlag für Hochschulschriften

Impressum / Imprint

Bibliografische Information der Deutschen Nationalbibliothek: Die Deutsche Nationalbibliothek verzeichnet diese Publikation in der Deutschen Nationalbibliografie; detaillierte bibliografische Daten sind im Internet über http://dnb.d-nb.de abrufbar.
Alle in diesem Buch genannten Marken und Produktnamen unterliegen warenzeichen-, marken- oder patentrechtlichem Schutz bzw. sind Warenzeichen oder eingetragene Warenzeichen der jeweiligen Inhaber. Die Wiedergabe von Marken, Produktnamen, Gebrauchsnamen, Handelsnamen, Warenbezeichnungen u.s.w. in diesem Werk berechtigt auch ohne besondere Kennzeichnung nicht zu der Annahme, dass solche Namen im Sinne der Warenzeichen- und Markenschutzgesetzgebung als frei zu betrachten wären und daher von jedermann benutzt werden dürften.

Bibliographic information published by the Deutsche Nationalbibliothek: The Deutsche Nationalbibliothek lists this publication in the Deutsche Nationalbibliografie; detailed bibliographic data are available in the Internet at http://dnb.d-nb.de.
Any brand names and product names mentioned in this book are subject to trademark, brand or patent protection and are trademarks or registered trademarks of their respective holders. The use of brand names, product names, common names, trade names, product descriptions etc. even without a particular marking in this works is in no way to be construed to mean that such names may be regarded as unrestricted in respect of trademark and brand protection legislation and could thus be used by anyone.

Coverbild / Cover image: www.ingimage.com

Verlag / Publisher:
Südwestdeutscher Verlag für Hochschulschriften
ist ein Imprint der / is a trademark of
OmniScriptum GmbH & Co. KG
Heinrich-Böcking-Str. 6-8, 66121 Saarbrücken, Deutschland / Germany
Email: info@svh-verlag.de

Herstellung: siehe letzte Seite /
Printed at: see last page
ISBN: 978-3-8381-3814-5

Zugl. / Approved by: Zurich, ETH, Diss. #20003, 2011

Copyright © 2014 OmniScriptum GmbH & Co. KG
Alle Rechte vorbehalten. / All rights reserved. Saarbrücken 2014

Table of Contents

SUMMARY	3
1 GENERAL INTRODUCTION	**7**
1.1 SPINAL CORD INJURY	7
1.2 LOCOMOTION AFTER SPINAL CORD INJURY	12
1.3 AIM OF THE PRESENT WORK	18
2 REHABILITATION IN SPINE AND SPINAL CORD TRAUMA	**20**
2.1 ABSTRACT	20
2.2 OBJECTIVE	21
2.3 INTRODUCTION	21
2.4 MATERIALS AND METHODS	22
2.5 RESULTS	25
2.6 CONCLUSIONS	29
2.7 KEY POINTS	30
2.8 ACKNOWLEDGEMENT	31
2.9 EVIDENTIARY TABLES	32
3 FUNCTIONAL WALKING AFTER INCOMPLETE SPINAL CORD INJURY – SHOULD THE 10 METER WALK TEST BE CURVY?	**43**
3.1 ABSTRACT	43
3.2 INTRODUCTION	44
3.3 METHODS	47
3.4 RESULTS	53
3.5 DISCUSSION	57
3.6 CONCLUSION	61
3.7 ACKNOWLEDGEMENT	62
4 INSTRUMENT VALIDITY AND RELIABILITY OF A CHOICE RESPONSE TIME TEST FOR INCOMPLETE SPINAL CORD INJURED SUBJECTS: RELATIONSHIP WITH FUNCTION	**63**
4.1 ABSTRACT	63
4.2 INTRODUCTION	64
4.3 METHODS	66
4.4 RESULTS	71
4.5 DISCUSSION	78
4.6 CONCLUSION	82
4.7 ACKNOWLEDGEMENT	82
5 MOTOR DEFICITS IN WELL-REHABILITATED PEOPLE WITH INCOMPLETE SPINAL CORD INJURY – A NEVER-ENDING STORY?	**83**
5.1 ABSTRACT	83
5.2 INTRODUCTION	84
5.3 METHODS	87
5.4 RESULTS	93
5.5 DISCUSSION	96
5.6 CONCLUSION	103

6 LOWER EXTREMITY STRENGTH TRAINING OUTPERFORMS ROBOT-ASSISTED GAIT TRAINING IN WALKING-RELATED OUTCOME MEASURES IN MODERATELY AMBULATING SUBJECTS WITH INCOMPLETE SPINAL CORD INJURY 104

6.1 ABSTRACT 104
6.2 INTRODUCTION 105
6.3 METHODS 108
6.4 RESULTS 119
6.5 DISCUSSION 123
6.6 CONCLUSION 130

7 EFFECTS OF ROBOT-ASSISTED GAIT TRAINING AND LOWER EXTREMITY STRENGTH TRAINING ON MOTOR EVOKED POTENTIALS AND RESPONSE TIMES OF THE LEG IN MODERATELY AMBULATING SUBJECTS WITH INCOMPLETE SPINAL CORD INJURY 131

7.1 ABSTRACT 131
7.2 INTRODUCTION 132
7.3 METHODS 135
7.4 RESULTS 137
7.5 DISCUSSION 141
7.6 CONCLUSION 144

8 PAIN ALLEVIATION AFTER ROBOT-ASSISTED GAIT TRAINING IN PATIENTS WITH INCOMPLETE SPINAL CORD INJURY 145

8.1 ABSTRACT 145
8.2 INTRODUCTION 146
8.3 METHODS 148
8.4 RESULTS 153
8.5 DISCUSSION 157
8.6 CONCLUSION 160
8.7 ACKNOWLEDGEMENT 160

9 GENERAL DISCUSSION 161

9.1 FIGURE OF EIGHT TEST 163
9.2 REACTION AND EXECUTION TEST 164

10 REFERENCES 166

11 ABBREVIATIONS 203

12 CURRICULUM VITAE 206

13 PUBLICATIONS 209

14 ACKNOWLEDGEMENT 210

Summary

Spinal cord injury is a diagnosis with a potentially high impact on the integrity of the person concerned. It causes destruction and demyelination of axonal pathways as well as segmental spinal circuitries and therefore affects conduction of sensory and motor signals across the lesion site. To help patients with spinal cord injury to deal with the consequences of these disruptions and to improve future outcome, a highly specific field of research has evolved. While in the past the potential for recovery after spinal cord injury was very limited, several new regeneration-inducing therapies are currently under investigation, and sophisticated rehabilitation methods have advanced. To properly monitor effectiveness of these therapies, it is therefore important that valid, reliable and responsive outcome measures are applied to assess changes in function of subjects with spinal cord injury. The responsiveness especially is an issue in ambulating patients with incomplete spinal cord injury, since this population tends to experience ceiling effects in established clinical assessments of function such as the ASIA motor score or the Walking Index for Spinal Cord Injury.

This work contributes to the expansion of knowledge in this field by investigating two new outcome measures that focus on adaptive walking and lower extremity response time. It furthermore delivers an overview of already existing and established outcome measures.

The Figure of Eight Test is a walking test that incorporates curve-walking and challenging situations like obstacles or cognitive distraction. It is a valid assessment tool in healthy subjects as well as subjects with incomplete spinal cord injury, and it adds information to the current gold standard, the 10m Walk Test, which focuses on straight, unobstructed walking. However, the 10m Walk Test is still superior in estimating functional ambulation performance.

The Reaction and Execution Test is a lower extremity response time test, which is performed in a standing position. Subjects have to move their leg as fast as possible to one of five buttons in response to respective flashing lights. The test showed good validity and reliability in patients with incomplete spinal cord injury and correlated significantly with several strength and ambulatory functional outcome measures. We furthermore combined the Reaction and Execution Test with transcranial magnetic stimulation and electromyography and demonstrated that well-recovered subjects with incomplete spinal cord injury still suffer from motor deficits, although they showed similar strength values compared to a matched able-bodied group. Apparently, response times might be a sensitive indicator of even slight deficits in motor function.

The last part of this work presents results of a training study, where the effects of task-specific locomotor training (performed as robot-assisted treadmill training) were compared with those of task-unspecific strength training. Thereby strength training led to greater improvements especially in walking tests, like the Figure of Eight Test, whereas neither intervention showed effects on response time. In the course of this study we also showed beneficial effects of robot-assisted gait training on pain intensity in subjects with incomplete spinal cord injury.

These results increase the current knowledge of motor function after incomplete spinal cord injury. The tests introduced above can be used to characterize remaining motor deficits to a higher degree compared to established measures. With rehabilitation in mind, the current gait-specific rehabilitation approach should be expanded to curve-walking and complemented by strength training. To evaluate the effectiveness of upcoming regeneration-inducing therapies after incomplete spinal cord injury, it is crucial to improve the sensitivity of current clinical assessment batteries by introducing additional outcome measures, such as those presented in this book.

Summary

1 General Introduction

1.1 Spinal cord injury

1.1.1 General information

The spinal cord together with the brain makes up the central nervous system. Thereby the spinal cord has three main functions. It receives and transmits efferent information from the brain to the periphery, it receives and transmits afferent information to the brain and it executes autonomic movements via its so-called central pattern generator (Dietz and Harkema, 2004). A lesion of the spinal cord by traumatic accidents or non-traumatic causes like tumors, infections or disc herniations can result in a wide range of physical and psychosocial problems. These problems can interfere with a person's personal health, feeling of well being and social interaction. However, depending on the density and location of the spinal lesion, the symptoms can vary greatly. A lesion of the cervical region of the cord usually affects all four limbs, trunk and pelvic organs, a condition referred to as tetraplegia, whilst injuries in the thoracic and lumbar regions lead to paraplegia. Furthermore, a spinal cord injury (SCI) must not always result in a life dependent on a wheelchair since neural transmission below the injury level can be affected to varying degrees. In about 50% of the cases, motor and/or sensory function is preserved below the lesion level (Wyndaele and Wyndaele, 2006); such an injury is termed incomplete, whilst the converse case (no sensory or motor function below the lesion) is called a complete injury. Aside from the primary damage of the spinal cord, further, secondary complications can be incurred through a series of biochemical and cellular processes internal to the body (Sekhon and Fehlings, 2001). Apart from the paralysis and sensory impairments, an SCI is often associated with additional issues like pain or social and economic difficulties. In Switzerland the incidence of SCI lies between 300-400 cases per year (Eberhard, 2004). This results in approximately 5 new SCI subjects per 100'000 inhabitants each year and that approximately corresponds to values given for other developed countries (Ackery et al., 2004; National Spinal Cord Injury Statistical Center Fact sheet, 2011).

To help patients with an SCI dealing with above-mentioned consequences, a highly specific field of rehabilitation has evolved. The goal of rehabilitation after SCI is to enable the person to resume a physically and functionally adequate lifestyle, and also to help the person integrating with his family, community and society. It therefore requires a comprehensive understanding of all different physiological and functional adaptations that occur with SCI and in the course of rehabilitation. It is therefore in the interest of SCI patients and also of the respective scientific community that progress of function is tracked using appropriate, valid and reliable clinical outcome measures. While in the past the potential for recovery after SCI was very limited, several new regeneration-inducing therapies are currently under investigation (Kwon et al., 2011a,b; Cadotte and Fehlings, 2011). To properly monitor the effectiveness of these therapies, clinical assessment tools become more important than ever and this work should contribute to the expansion of knowledge in this field.

1.1.2 Classification of Spinal Cord Injury

An SCI is usually classified by level and completeness of the injury. The assessment of spinal cord function is done according to the "International Standards for Neurological Classification of Spinal Cord Injury", as established by the American Spinal Injury Association (ASIA, Marino et al., 2003). Motor function of specific segments of the upper and lower extremity is tested in 10 key muscles on each side of the body and graded from 0-5 (Tab. 1.1). Sensory function is quantified by testing the sensitivity of light touch and pin prick in all dermatomes at defined key points on both body sides. The sensitivity is scored as 0 (absent), 1 (impaired) or 2 (normal).

The International Standards provide motor and sensory scores, unilateral levels of motor and sensory lesion, as well as the neurological level of lesion, which is defined as the most caudal segment of the spinal cord where normal motor and sensory function is preserved. Importantly, the neurological level is not congruent with the skeletal level, which refers to the level at which the greatest vertebral damage is found by radiographic examination after traumatic lesions.

Particularly in the thoracic and lumbar spine, these levels deviate considerably due to the fact that the spinal cord ends approximately at the level of the second lumbar vertebra. Finally, all information of the International Standards can be combined and results in the description of 5 categories reflecting the severity or completeness of

Score	Description
0	Total paralysis
1	Palpable or visible contraction
2	Active movement, full range of motion with gravity eliminated
3	Active movement, full range of motion against gravity
4	Active movement, full range of motion against moderate resistance
5	Active movement, full range of motion against full resistance

Tab. 1.1: Assessment of muscle strength according to the American Spinal Injury Association.

the injury. This is named the ASIA Impairment Scale (AIS, Tab. 1.2).

However, despite over 20 years of experience in applying the International Standards (and its predecessor the Frankel scale) there are several limitations of this measure. The motor score according to ASIA for example has an ordinal data structure. The lacking sensitivity due to ceiling effects has therefore been criticized in several studies (Herbison et al., 1996; Noreau and Vachon, 1998). Furthermore, the ASIA motor score may for example not be sensitive to subtle weakness or impairment in movement velocity that could be a result of SCI. These would have to be detected otherwise and there are several established outcome measures of motor function for people with SCI (a detailed overview can be found in chapter 2).

Grade	Completeness	Functional impairment
A	Complete	No sensory or motor function is preserved in the sacral segments S4-S5
B	Incomplete	Sensory but not motor function is preserved below the neurological level and includes the sacral segments S4-S5
C	Incomplete	Motor function is preserved below the neurological level, and more than half of key muscles below the neurological level have a muscle grade less than 3 (Grades 0-2)
D	Incomplete	Motor function is preserved below the neurological level, and at least half of key muscles below the neurological level have a muscle grade greater than or equal to 3
E	n.a.	Sensory and motor function is normal

Tab. 1.2: Classification of spinal cord injury according to the American Spinal Injury Association Impairment Scale (Marino et al., 2003).

1.1.3 Clinical assessments in patients with spinal cord injury

As outlined in chapter 1.1.1, outcome measures are important tools in clinical as well as scientific settings. Adapted from Steeves et al., 2007, 3 main groups of outcome measures are described below:

(1) Assessment of neurological connectivity of the spinal cord, without considering the ability of the patient to functionally use these connections. An example for such an outcome measure would be the neurological scoring, as described in chapter 1.1.2. It also includes assessments of neurological capacity that are independent

of the environment (e.g. electrophysiological recordings or imaging assessments).

(2) Assessments of an individual's level of participation in societal activities. As these will not be discussed in this book, further information can be found elsewhere (Hill et al., 2009).

(3) Assessment of activities of daily living. An example would be the Spinal Cord Independence Measure (SCIM, Itzkovich et al., 2007). Functional evaluations may be more adequate to detect clinically meaningful changes in the functional capacity of a patient, but they also depend on motivation, rehabilitation, fitness and other factors. Therefore, any change in a person's functional capacity after SCI may be due to adaptive changes within and/or without the central nervous system. Further examples are outcome measures of ambulatory function, as illustrated in chapter 1.2.4.

1.2 Locomotion after spinal cord injury

1.2.1 Control of locomotion in general

Walking and thus interacting with a constantly changing environment is a normal daily activity for most people. It is not necessary to consciously think how the legs should be moved, it happens 'automatically'. However, this might not longer be the case when walking function becomes impaired (e.g. after an incomplete spinal cord injury [iSCI]).

Gait is assumed to be controlled hierarchically, where higher levels of the central nervous system control adaptive processes of gait, while lower levels carry out detailed monitoring and regulation of the response execution (Shumway-Cook and Woollacott, 2001). At the top of this hierarchy is a supraspinal locomotor network that consists of frontal cortex, basal ganglia, brain stem tegmentum and cerebellum. This network controls adaptive regulation, like initiation and termination of gait and changes of velocity and direction (Nutt et al., 2011). At the bottom of the hierarchy is the spinal cord. Nevertheless, it is suggested that some essential requirements for motor control of gait are already partially coordinated at spinal level (Poppele and Bosco, 2003) by the central pattern generator. This is a spinal network that generates reciprocal rhythmic activation patterns of flexor and extensor muscles for simple locomotion, even without any input from the brain (Grillner, 2002; Dietz, 2003). It exists also in humans and with intact sensory input, it is capable of generating these motor bursts autonomously (Duysens and van de Crommert, 1998). Accordingly, experiments using transcranial magnetic stimulation (TMS) have provided evidence that the excitability of corticospinal pathways to leg and arm muscles is modulated as a function of the gait cycle and that corticospinal drive contributes directly to the activation of involved muscles during uncomplicated treadmill walking (Barthélemy and Nielsen, 2010). The treadmill thereby delivers peripheral feedback (e.g. via peripheral reflexes or proprioception). Indeed, proprioceptive feedback from muscle afferents seems to be essential for the regulation of basic locomotor patterns. The central pattern generator as well as reflex mechanisms are controlled by the above-mentioned supraspinal locomotor network (for review and more details, see: Dietz, 2003; Nutt et al., 2011).

1.2.2 Implications for patients with incomplete spinal cord injury

Since an SCI can lead to disturbed descending control and ascending feedback, patients with iSCI strongly depend on visual input to compensate for proprioceptive deficits and impaired balance (van Hedel and Dietz, 2010). Furthermore, they require additional attentional demands while walking (Lajoie et al., 1999). These factors might contribute to the higher risk of falling in this population (up to 75%, Brotherton et al., 2007), even when some of these patients walk long distances and do not need assistive devices in their everyday life. There is further evidence that even in well-recovered SCI subjects, small deficiencies in walking-related function persist, which remain undetected by established clinical walking tests. A recent publication showed for example that maximal movement velocity was impaired and related well to corticospinal tract integrity, while impairments in strength as quantified with the ASIA motor score did not correlate well. Furthermore, around 50-60% of variability in walking speed could be explained by maximal movement velocity (Wirth et al., 2008a). Maximal movement velocity seems to be an important factor, especially since a timely correct foot placement plays an important role in quickly adjusting the locomotor pattern to changing external demands (Chen et al., 1994). Furthermore, the double-support duration during gait is increased even in well-recovered iSCI subjects (van Hedel et al., 2005a).

1.2.3 Recovery of locomotion after incomplete spinal cord injury

Independent from time after lesion, age at time of injury or severity of the SCI, restoration of motor function including walking ability is given a high priority by people with SCI (Ditunno et al., 2008a). Patients with iSCI often show substantial recovery of ambulatory function. Dobkin et al. showed that 92% of patients with iSCI with little motor function below the neurological level (AIS grade C) at 2 months post injury were able to walk independently half a year later (Dobkin et al., 2007). From the same study, it is known that 100% of patients with iSCI with strong motor function below the neurological level at 2 months post injury (AIS grade D) regained their walking ability half a year later (Dobkin et al., 2007). This is in line with the continuous increase of ASIA motor scores during the course of recovery after iSCI (Waters et al., 1994a,b). The plethora of processes that lead to these improvements is not yet very well understood, however, mainly three categories of mechanisms are currently in focus, adaptation/compensation, regeneration/repair and reorganization of neuronal circuits (Curt et al., 2008) and those will shortly be discussed subsequently.

Adaptation/compensation

In clinical rehabilitation, recovery of sensorimotor function is generally achieved by adaptation (e.g. application of an assistive device, like an orthosis) and compensation (using healthy structures to compensate for damaged ones, e.g. training of new muscle synergies) (Curt et al., 2004). Compensatory mechanisms, which do not influence the central nervous system itself, extensively contribute to this recovery. These mechanisms involve changes at the level of motor behavior as well as changes in motor units and they are supported by training (Curt et al., 2008).

Regeneration/repair

In contrast to the peripheral nervous system, neurons of the central nervous system normally fail to regenerate their axons after injury in mammals. This failure is largely due to inhibitory molecules, and additionally, reactive astrocytes at the site of injury form a glial scar. Numerous strategies to overcome these barriers to regeneration are currently being investigated (for review, see: Kwon et al, 2011a,b; Cadotte and Fehlings, 2011).

Reorganization of neuronal circuits

Neural plasticity can be defined as the compensation of damaged structures by reorganization of preserved structures. It can be influenced by training (Curt et al., 2008) and also occurs spontaneously and is mediated by strengthening or weakening of pre-existing circuits, as well as by the formation of new circuits through collateral sprouting (Bareyre et al., 2004). After iSCI, plasticity occurs at cortical, subcortical and spinal levels (Ding et al., 2005). For recovery of ambulation after SCI, especially plasticity in the central pattern generator at spinal level is hypothesized to be important (Harkema, 2001). The specific response of the human spinal cord to sensory information related to locomotion-specific training indicates the potential recovery of walking after SCI

(Behrman and Harkema, 2000).

1.2.4 Assessment of locomotor function after spinal cord injury

Well established measures of locomotor function are the 10m Walk Test (10MWT) (van Hedel et al., 2005b), the revised version of the Walking Index for Spinal Cord Injury (WISCI II) (Ditunno and Ditunno, 2001) and the Spinal Cord Independence Measure (SCIM, mobility part) (Itzkovich et al., 2007). The ASIA motor score of certain lower extremity muscles has been shown to correlate with walking speed (Scivoletto and Di Donna, 2009; Yang et al., 2011) and together with age and sensory scores, the probability of independent walking can be predicted early after traumatic injury (van Middendorp et al., 2011). In addition, locomotor outcome after SCI can be predicted using neurophysiology, e.g. somatosensory evoked potentials to assess afferent impulse conductivity of the spinal tract (Curt and Dietz, 1997) or motor evoked potentials (MEP) to assess corticospinal tract function (Curt et al., 1998). Finally, locomotor function after SCI can be investigated on a muscular level (by electromyographic recordings [EMG], e.g. Dietz and Harkema, 2004) or on a biomechanical level (by kinematic [Krawetz and Nance, 1996] or kinetic analyses [Melis et al., 1999]).

One drawback of current clinical walking assessments is their focus on straight unobstructed walking and their inability to assess the capacity of adapting to environmental constraints, which should be the final goal of rehabilitation (Ladouceur et al., 2003). This is especially the case in well-recovered patients, where current outcome measures show ceiling effects. Additionally, improved outcome measures could also help identifying changes induced by rehabilitation more specifically. The work done in this work tries to fill part of that gap.

1.3 Aim of the present work

The assessment of the recovery of motor function is an important issue in the rehabilitation of patients with iSCI, both for the evaluation and comparison of established and new therapeutical approaches. This also includes walking-related outcomes. It is therefore important that valid, reliable and responsive measurement tools are applied to assess changes in the functional ability in iSCI subjects. Especially for well-recovered subjects available tools are limited due to ceiling effects. The general aim of this work is to give an overview over already existing outcome measures, to evaluate 2 newly developed assessment tools and to test their performance in a training intervention with iSCI patients.

The specific topics are the following:
- Review of the most clinically relevant outcome measures of motor function for rehabilitating patients with SCI (chapter 2)
- Investigation of a newly developed walking test that incorporates curve-walking and challenging situations in able-bodied and iSCI subjects (chapter 3)
- Investigation of a newly developed lower extremity response time test in able-bodied and iSCI subjects (chapters 4 and 5)
- Investigation of the importance of task-specificity of training on

outcome of walking-related function in iSCI subjects (chapters 6 and 7)
- Influence of robot-assisted gait training on short-term and longitudinal development of pain in iSCI subjects (chapter 8)

2 Rehabilitation in Spine and Spinal Cord Trauma

Published in the journal *Spine*: Labruyère R, Agarwala A, Curt A. Rehabilitation in spine and spinal cord trauma. Spine. 2010;35(21 Suppl):S259-62.

2.1 Abstract

Study Design: Systematic Review

Objectives: To define the optimal time for initiation of rehabilitation and review the most clinically relevant outcome measures of upper and lower limb motor function of the rehabilitating spinal cord injured patient utilizing a systematic review and expert opinion.

Summary of Background Data: Comprehensive rehabilitation programs are required for patients after SCI as early as feasible. In a dedicated spinal cord injury rehabilitation setting, effective treatment and proper monitoring of spontaneous and rehabilitation-based motor function improvements by means of appropriate, valid, reliable and internationally accepted clinical assessment tools is warranted.

Methods: Focused questions on key topics in rehabilitation of the spinal cord injured patient were defined by a panel of spine trauma surgeons. A keyword literature search for pertinent articles was conducted using multiple databases. Suitable articles were screened and the quality of evidence was graded and tabulated. Based on the evidence and expert opinion, recommendations were composed and rated as strong or weak.

Results: The outcome measures literature search yielded a total of

1251 abstracts. Out of these 86 articles were studied in detail. One high quality study was found with three articles referring to it. Furthermore, there were 19 moderate quality, 39 low quality and 25 very low quality studies. The timing literature search yielded 508 abstracts of which 3 articles focused on the question and were all graded as low quality.

Conclusions: For general motor function, assessing the ASIA motor score and the Spinal Cord Independence Measure III is strongly recommended. The ASIA motor score is also useful in assessing upper and lower extremity motor function. For ambulatory function a timed walk test like the 10 Meter Walk test in combination with the Walking Index for Spinal Cord Injury II is strongly recommended. Early rehabilitation, defined as within 30 days of injury, improves outcome and recovery for spinal cord trauma patients.

2.2 Objective

The goal of this article is to give an overview of two important topics in rehabilitation of the spinal cord injured patient. First, we identified clinically relevant outcome measures of upper and lower limb motor function. Second, we reviewed the effect of timing of initiation of rehabilitation in spinal cord injury (SCI). A systematic review was performed to combine evidence in the literature and expert opinion from the Spine Trauma Study Group.

2.3 Introduction

Comprehensive rehabilitation programs are required for patients after SCI as early as feasible. In several countries, the time point of admission to an active inpatient SCI-specific rehabilitation setting, at which rehabilitation is perceived as restitutio ad optimum, can exceed thirty days. In this period, effective treatment and proper monitoring of spontaneous and rehabilitation-based motor function improvements is lacking, but would be essential for an optimal outcome of rehabilitation and the translation of experimental interventions in the clinical setting.

In the interest of SCI patients and also for scientific reasons, it is desirable that progress of motor function is monitored using appropriate, valid, reliable and internationally accepted clinical assessment tools.

To facilitate this, it is the aim of this systematic review to give an overview of common outcome measures for the assessment of motor function and to highlight the importance of an early admission to rehabilitation.

2.4 Materials and Methods

The systematic review was focused on the following research questions:
- What assessment instruments should be collected to evaluate the outcome of upper and lower limb motor function after SCI?
- What is the optimal timing for initiation of active rehabilitation following acute SCI?

A comprehensive literature search was conducted using MEDLINE, EMBASE and the Cochrane Database of Systematic reviews.

Inclusion criteria:
- Articles published between 1980 and May 2009
- Articles in English
- Traumatic SCI
- Adult age group (18+ years)
- Randomized controlled trials, cohort studies, case-control studies, cross-sectional studies, case series, review articles

Exclusion criteria:
1. Case reports
2. Pediatric age group
3. Mixed pathology

For papers addressing outcome measures, studies about the general function of spinal cord injured subjects were only included if they specifically addressed motor function items. Articles about the Functional Independence Measure (FIM), for example, were only considered if the subscale motor FIM was separately mentioned.

The abstracts of all articles that matched the search terms and inclusion/exclusion criteria were reviewed and full text versions of suitable articles were obtained. For question two, one article was translated from Chinese and able to be included (Deng et al., 2004). It was then checked whether these articles could make a contribution to answering the research question. If so, their reference lists were hand-searched for further relevant literature, which was then also added to the final list of papers.

For papers discussing outcome measures, the results were divided into five subgroups: general motor function – upper extremity motor function – lower extremity motor function – wheelchair – ambulation. Results addressing more then one of the above-mentioned subgroups were allocated in the general motor function subgroup. Papers were tabulated as evidentiary tables for both research questions.

This review covers the following grading of the quality of the literature (Mace et al., 2008; Schunemann et al., 2006):
High quality: Randomized controlled trials, meta-analysis of randomized controlled trials; Moderate quality: Downgraded high quality studies (due to serious limitations or inconsistencies), non-randomized trials, prospective cohort studies; Low quality: Retrospective observational, retrospective cohort, and case control studies; Very low quality: Case series, case reports, reviews, other. Some designs didn't fit into this scheme and were graded individually. Ambispective studies were classified as retrospective, since usually an essential part of the data was gained retrospectively. To delineate cohort studies from case series, we defined that a cohort should at least cover 30 subjects.

2.5 Results

2.5.1 Question #1 - Assessment Instruments:

The literature search resulted in a total of 1251 abstracts. Out of these, 86 relevant articles were looked at in detail. One high quality study was found, and three articles were referring to it. Furthermore, there were 19 moderate quality, 39 low quality and 25 very low quality studies.

General motor function

37 articles were found with information about general motor function (Table 2.1). They give an overview of most motor function outcome measures actually applied in SCI rehabilitation. Among these, especially three measures stand out. The American Spinal Injury Association (ASIA) Motor Score (AMS), the FIM and the Spinal Cord Independence Measure (SCIM) are used worldwide and all but two articles are referring to at least one of these three measures. So there seems to be some consensus on the instruments used for measurement of general motor function. The AMS is a widely accepted and applied measure to quickly assess muscle strength. It is part of the International Standards for Neurological Classification of SCI (Marino et al., 2003) and should be tracked separately for upper and lower extremity (Alexander et al., 2009; Marino et al., 2004; Steeves et al., 2007). It generally shows no age-related (Cifu et al., 1999) and gender-related (Greenwald et al., 2001) differences. However, assessment of AMS alone is not enough to reflect an SCI subject's function (Dvorak et al., 2005). The FIM is the gold standard in measuring functional independence in subjects with

neurologic disorders. However, it was not specifically designed for the SCI population. The SCIM fills that gap and is therefore superior to the FIM in its use on SCI population (Catz et al., 1997). The current version of SCIM, the SCIM III, is a valid and reliable tool to assess the functional capacity of SCI subjects and can be used in a clinical as well as a scientific setting (Itzkovich et al., 2007). In assessing independence in SCI subjects, SCIM should therefore always be favored over FIM, as endorsed by Furlan et al. (Furlan et al., 2011).

Upper extremity motor function
There were 17 articles with information about upper extremity motor function (Table 2.2). These articles contain a broad range of outcome measures, mainly dividable into three subgroups: "Assessment of hand and arm function (ADL)", "Assessment of hand an arm function (physiology)" and "Prediction of hand and arm function". For the subgroup "Assessment of hand and arm function (ADL)", there are at least 6 different tests that partly overlap, and none of those is clearly superior to the others. Also there does not seem to be any consensus on which test to preferably use. For research use, the Grasp and Release Test (GRT) seems adequate (Mulcahey et al., 2007). A promising new tool is the Graded and Redefined Assessment of Strength, Sensibility and Prehension (GRASSP), which is actually being tested for validity and reliability (Alexander et al., 2009). All in all more studies are needed to clearly depict a standard measurement of the ADL hand and arm function. For the subgroup "Assessment of hand an arm function

(physiology)" there only was scarce literature evidence. For the subgroup "Prediction of hand and arm function" again the AMS seems to be of value (Marino et al., 1998; Rudhe and van Hedel, 2009; Yavuz et al., 1998). It can be complemented by Manual Muscle Testing (MMT) (Rudhe and van Hedel, 2009; Jacquemin et al., 2004; van Tuijl et al., 2002) or dynamometry (Jacquemin et al., 2004; van Tuijl et al., 2002; Schwartz et al., 1992).

Lower extremity motor function
There were 2 articles specifically looking at outcome measures regarding lower extremity motor function without addressing ambulation (Table 2.3). Lim et al. showed that the surface electromyography-based Voluntary Response Index (VRI) could be used to quantitatively measure SCI severity in terms of voluntary motor control disruption (Lim et al., 2005). Lynch et al. demonstrated that the Functional Reach Test (FRT) could roughly measure differences among levels of SCI (Lynch et al., 1998).

Wheelchair
There were 4 articles regarding wheelchair motor function (Table 2.4). These articles all describe different tests to evaluate mobility in wheelchair-dependent SCI subjects. All of these tests assess wheelchair skills, whereas one also measures transfer abilities of the subject (Harvey et al., 1998), and another one specific handling of the wheelchair (like use of the footrests or folding of the wheelchair) (Kirby et al., 2002).

Ambulation

There were 26 articles looking at ambulatory function (Table 2.5). Most addressed outcome measures in this subgroup were the walk tests over different distances (50 feet, 8 meters and 10 meters) and the Walking Index for Spinal Cord Injury (WISCI) as a test to quantify the use of assistive devices. The 6 Minutes Walk Test (6MWT) does not seem to assess a different domain of mobility compared to the 50 Foot Walk Test (50FWT, Barbeau et al., 2007). Prediction of walking recovery can be done neurophysiologically, for example with somatosensory evoked potentials (SEP, Curt and Dietz, 1997), motor evoked potentials (MEP, Scivoletto and Di Donna, 2009) or delayed plantar response (DPR, Scivoletto et Di Donna, 2009). Also the AMS can be of prognostic value (Scivoletto and Di Donna, 2009).

2.5.2 Question #2 - Optimal Timing:

The literature search yielded 508 articles of which 3 suitable articles addressed the question and were reviewed in detail (Table 2.6). All three articles were designed as retrospective cohorts and therefore graded as low quality. One article, which was translated from Chinese, divided patients into two groups based on immediate rehabilitation admission and greater than 6 months after SCI prior to rehabilitation admission (Deng et al., 2004). The second article created 3 groups for time to initiation of rehabilitation as within 2 weeks of injury, 2 weeks to 6 months, and greater than 6 months (Sumida et al., 2001). The third article reviewed created matched triads based on the ASIA Impairment Scale (AIS), lesion level, age and sex grouped as short time to admission for active rehabilitation (less than 30 days), medium (31 to 60 days), and long (greater than 60 days) (Scivoletto et al., 2005). All articles used similar outcome measures of Barthel Index (BI), AIS and FIM scores to assess outcome.

In all three articles, earlier admission to rehabilitation after acute SCI showed greater improvement in activities of daily living (ADL) by standard outcome measurements. In the study with matched triads, considered the highest quality study in this review, the short time to admission to rehabilitation group outperformed the other two groups in ADL as measured by BI and the mobility scores (WISCI) were significantly better (Scivoletto et al., 2005). As motor recovery was similar between groups in this study, it was felt this was not a confounding factor for improved outcomes in the early rehabilitation patients. In the other two studies, the earlier rehabilitation groups had better motor recovery (Deng et al., 2004; Sumida et al., 2001). It is important to note that these studies were performed in dedicated SCI rehabilitation centers, where kind, length and intensity of rehabilitation are designed to meet SCI patients' needs. However, there is only scarce literature about the optimal length and intensity of rehabilitation for SCI patients and high quality studies are needed to elucidate this scientifically and economically important issue.

2.6 Conclusions

This systematic review was performed to answer two questions and make recommendations for rehabilitation of the acute SCI patient.

- What assessment instruments should be collected to evaluate the outcome of upper and lower limb motor function after SCI?
- What is the optimal timing for initiation of active rehabilitation following acute SCI?

The Spine Trauma Study Group gives a strong recommendation for assessing general motor function in SCI patients with the AMS and the SCIM III. For ambulatory function, walk tests as reviewed above in combination with the WISCI II are strongly recommended. A strong recommendation for early initiation of rehabilitation after SCI is made based on this review. Early rehab is defined as within 30 days. The criteria for admission should be the ability to participate in active rehab and admission should be to a dedicated SCI rehabilitation center.

2.7 Key Points

- For general motor function, the ASIA motor score and the Spinal Cord Independence Measure III are strongly recommended. The ASIA motor score is also useful in assessing upper extremity motor function.
- For ambulatory function a timed walk test in combination with the Walking Index for Spinal Cord Injury II is strongly recommended.
- Initiation of rehabilitation in a dedicated spinal cord injury rehabilitation center within 30 days of acute trauma leads to improved outcomes in spinal cord injured patients.

2.8 Acknowledgement

R. Labruyère was paid from grants of the International Spinal Research Trust (Clinical Initiative Stage 2, London, Great Britain) and the EMDO Foundation (Zurich, Switzerland).

2.9 Evidentiary tables

First Author	Year	Design (total no. of subjects)	Outcome Measures	Grading	Relevant Findings
Aito et al.	2007	Retrosp. Cohort (82)	AMS/FIM/WISCI	Low	FIM and WISCI scores are significantly influenced by spasticity and age in subjects with central cord syndrome.
Alexander et al.	2009	Review	Several	Very low	The AMS should be tracked separately for upper and lower limb muscles. MMT is probably more reliable than myometry, but maybe not sensitive to changes in the upper range of strength. A combination of EMG, MEP and SEP might be of importance in predicting functional clinical benefit. The VRI needs further validation. FIM and SCIM are reliable and they are valid unlike MBI and QIF. FIM might not reflect functional recovery in SCI. SCIM and QIF are recommended for further development. GRT is reliable, GRASSP is currently being tested on reliability and validity. For ambulation, WISCI and 10MWT are the most valid and clinically useful tests, FIM-L is least recommended.
Amsters et al.	2005	Retrosp. Cohort (84)	FIM	Low	Motor FIM and MAIDS change over the years after discharge from the rehabilitation center.
Beninato et al.	2004	Case Series (20)	FIM/MMT	Very low	Key muscles measured by MMT can be identified relative to motor FIM tasks.
Calancie et al.	2004a	Retrosp. Cohort (229)	Reflex/EMG	Low	Tendon response amplitude and reflex spread can sensitively indicate preserved supraspinal control over lower limb musculature in acute SCI.
Calancie et al.	2004b	Retrosp. Cohort (229)	EMG	Low	EMG can be used to assess the recovery of voluntary movement after acute SCI, but large inter-individual differences can be seen.

First Author	Year	Design (total no. of subjects)	Outcome Measures	Grading	Relevant Findings
Catz et al.	2007	Retrosp. Cohort (425)	SCIM	Low	Scores of the motor SCIM III seem to be a reliable representation of independence after SCI.
Catz et al.	2004	Retrosp. Cohort (79)	SCI-ARMI	Low	SCI-ARMI can be used to assess changes in functional ability. SCIM II scores correlate highly with AMS.
Catz et al.	2001	Case Series (28)	SCIM	Very low	The Catz-Itzkovich SCIM is superior to the original SCIM and should supersede it. It correlates significantly with the FIM.
Catz et al.	1997	Retrosp. Cohort (30)	SCIM/FIM	Low	The SCIM is superior to the FIM in assessing changes of function in SCI subjects.
Cifu et al.	1999	Retrosp. Cohort (375)	AMS/FIM	Low	There are no age-related differences in AMS and motor FIM at acute care and inpatient rehabilitation admission, but improvement over time is better in younger patients.
Curt et al.	2008	Retrosp. Cohort (460)	AMS/MEP/SEP	Low	Protocols combining neurological, functional, and spinal conductivity measures are required to distinguish between the effects of compensation, neural plasticity and repair mechanisms of damaged spinal tracts on recovery.
Curt et al.	1998	Prosp. Cohort (70)	AMS/MEP	Moderate	MEP and AMS are related to outcome of ambulatory capacity and hand function in SCI patients.
Dahlberg et al.	2003	Retrosp. Cohort (121)	FIM	Low	The walking/wheelchair locomotion item of the motor FIM lacks sensitivity in the chronic phase of SCI due to its ceiling effect. No significant difference between para- and tetraplegia in motor FIM score. There was also no age-dependency.
Dvorak et al.	2005	Retrosp. Cohort (70)	AMS/FIM	Low	The assessment of AMS in SCI subjects is not enough to obtain an overview of the function and outcomes in this population.
Ellaway et al.	2007	Review	AMS/MEP	Very low	The assessment of MEPs can compensate for the shortcoming of the AMS measurement regarding the thoracic myotomes.

First Author	Year	Design (total no. of subjects)	Outcome Measures	Grading	Relevant Findings
Fisher et al.	2005	Retrosp. Cohort (70)	AMS/FIM	Low	In complete SCI subjects, changes in AMS over time were low and reflected local recovery only.
Greenwald et al.	2001	Retrosp. Cohort (1074)	AMS/FIM	Low	There were no gender related differences in motor FIM and AMS on discharge compared to admission.
Haisma et al.	2008	Prosp. Cohort (176)	FIM	Moderate	Changes in motor FIM are associated with peak power output.
Harness et al.	2008	Prosp. Controlled Trial (29)	AMS	Moderate	There was a correlation between gains in AMS and number of hours of intense exercise in chronic SCI subjects.
Itzkovich et al.	2007	Retrosp. Cohort (425)	FIM/SCIM	Low	SCIM III is a valid and reliable measure for the functional assessment of SCI patients and can be used in a clinical setting and for research in a multi-cultural setup.
Itzkovich et al.	2003	Prosp. Case Series (28)	SCIM	Low	The rate of agreement between two interviewers for motor SCIM II items was 35% - 96%, but in most items not below 63%.
Itzkovich et al.	2002	Retrosp. Cohort (202)	FIM/SCIM	Low	Validity and reliability of the SCIM II are confirmed. But some items still need to be rephrased or removed.
Kirshblum et al.	2004	Retrosp. Cohort (987)	AMS	Low	58% of incomplete SCI subjects improved in AMS from 1 to 5 years post injury compared to 27% of complete SCI subjects. In neither group there were significant changes in motor level.
Lawton et al.	2006	Retrosp. Cohort (647)	FIM	Low	Results from motor FIM should not be compared from country to country. This can only be done after a fit to the Rasch model, but with a loss of clinical important items.
Lazar et al.	1989	Retrosp. Cohort (78)	AMS/MBI	Low	The AMS is a useful tool in predicting function during rehabilitation, but it shows difficulties in predicting ambulatory function. The AMS did not correlate with the mobility subscore of the MBI.
Lim et al.	2004	Case Control (19)	VRI	Low	The VRI is able to distinguish healthy from incomplete SCI subjects, it can characterize individual changes among incomplete SCI subjects and can track changes over time in motor control.

First Author	Year	Design (total no. of subjects)	Outcome Measures	Grading	Relevant Findings
Marino et al.	2004	Retrosp. Cohort (4338)	AMS/FIM	Low	Use of separate ASIA UEMS and LEMS can better predict motor FIM compared to the use of the total AMS.
McKinley et al.	2007	Retrosp. Cohort (175)	FIM	Low	There are differences in motor FIM at admission for people with different SCI clinical syndromes (best scores for patients with cauda equina syndrome and worst scores for patients with central cord syndrome).
Middleton et al.	2006	Prosp. Cohort (43)	5-AML/FIM	Moderate	The 5-AML items complement the motor FIM regarding the assessment of motor requirements outside of the rehabilitation center. They were shown to be valid and responsive.
Scivoletto et al.	2006	Retrosp. Cohort (117)	AMS/WISCI	Low	When comparing early to late admission to the rehabilitation center, WISCI and AMS develop similarly in incomplete SCI subjects.
Sipski et al.	2004	Retrosp. Cohort (14433)	AMS/FIM	Low	When subjects are divided in subgroups according to their level of lesion, there partly are gender related differences in motor FIM and AMS.
Steeves et al.	2007	Review	Several	Very low	Separate assessment of UEMS and LEMS is recommended. Dependent upon level and severity of SCI, different rehabilitation efficacy thresholds for AMS are defined. EMG, SEP and MEP provide quantitative data for assessing spinal conductivity and they can be performed on unresponsive subjects. WISCI, TUG, 10MWT and 6MWT are recommended for assessment of ambulatory function. For upper extremity function, there is no consensus on what outcome measure is currently recommendable. For SCI subjects SCIM is considered superior to FIM.
Sumida et al.	2001	Retrosp. Cohort (123)	AMS/FIM/MMR	Low	Outcome of MMR, FIM and AMS depend on time of admission to the rehabilitation center.
Taricco et al.	2000	Prosp. Cohort (100)	VFM	Moderate	VFM is a valid and reliable tool to screen SCI subjects for functional status and impact of rehabilitation.

First Author	Year	Design (total no. of subjects)	Outcome Measures	Grading	Relevant Findings
Tooth et al.	2003	Retrosp. Cohort (167)	FIM	Low	The improvement in FIM score over a 5-year interval is almost only due to an improvement in motor FIM score.
Wirth et al.	2008b	Retrosp. Cohort (100)	AMS/SCIM	Low	SCIM II is responsive to functional changes in subjects with a persistent complete SCI. It can further develop even if AMS persists.

Table 2.1: Evidentiary table – general motor function

First Author	Year	Design (total no. of subjects)	Outcome Measures	Grading	Conclusion
Curt et al.	1996a	Retrosp. Cohort (69)	SEP	Low	Assessment of SEP can predict the outcome of hand function.
Curt et al.	1996b	Retrosp. Cohort (41)	MCAP/NCV	Low	Neurography can be of prognostic value in cervical SCI to predict the outcome of hand function.
Dahlgren et al.	2007	Retrosp. Cohort (55)	KBS	Low	The KBS is useful for assessing daily activities in cervical SCI subjects, but its clinical application is limited due to problems with the weight scheme.
Hol et al.	2007	Prosp. Cohort (30)	6MAT	Moderate	The 6MAT as a tool for the assessment of cardiovascular fitness shows acceptable values for reliability and validity. It further needs to be tested for responsiveness.
Jacobs et al.	2003	Prosp. Cohort (43)	AWaNT	Moderate	AWAnT is a reliable tool to assess upper extremity muscular power in subjects with complete paraplegia.
Jacquemin et al.	2004	Prosp. Cohort (55)	Myometer/MMT	Moderate	Quantitative hand strength measurement with a dynamometer and MMT may allow for earlier diagnosis of secondary neurologic complications and for monitoring neurologic recovery.
Marino et al.	1998	Retrosp. Cohort (154)	AMS/CUE/FIM	Low	The CUE shows good values for homogeneity, reliability and validity. It further needs to be tested for sensitivity. CUE was superior to UEMS in predicting motor FIM scores.

2. Rehabilitation in Spine and Spinal Cord Trauma

First Author	Year	Design (total no. of subjects)	Outcome Measures	Grading	Conclusion
Mulcahey et al.	2007	Review	Several	Very low	Most common hand function tests are advised against due to limitations in their use with tetraplegics. To build evidence for interventions, one or a battery of the following tests should be applied: CUE, MCS, SHFT or THAQ. The GRT is recommended for scientific use.
Post et al.	2006	Prosp. Cohort (67)	GRT/VLT-SV	Moderate	The VLT-SV is a reliable and valid test to assess hand/arm function in tetraplegics.
Rudhe et al.	2009	Case Series (29)	AMS/MMT/SCIM	Very low	SCIM III scores correlated well with UEMS and MMT. Especially its self-care category reflects upper extremity performance in tetraplegics.
Schwartz et al.	1992	Prosp. Cohort (122)	Myometer/MMT	Moderate	Myometry seems to be more specific than MMT.
Sisto et al.	2007	Review	Dynamometry	Very low	Reliability of hand-held dynamometry is strongly dependent the respective testing procedure. It is particularly necessary that the examiner has enough strength. A drawback of this method is the limited range of motion tested. Isometric dynamometers are not suitable for bedside testing.
Sollerman et al.	1995	Prosp. Cohort (59)	SHFT	Moderate	The SHFT correlated well with a common disability rating and with the international classification of the patient's arm. It is reliable and reproducible.
Spooren et al.	2008	Prosp. Cohort (92)	FIM/GRT/QIF/VLT	Moderate	Motor incomplete SCI subjects achieve higher arm hand skilled performance than those with a motor complete lesion. To further optimize therapy, it may be necessary to monitor the outcome of hand function during rehabilitation phase.
Spooren et al.	2006	Prosp. Cohort (60)	FIM/GRT/QIF/VLT	Moderate	The VLT is responsive for the assessment of hand function of cervical SCI subjects. Its responsiveness is significantly correlated to the GRT, but not to FIM and QIF.

First Author	Year	Design (total no. of subjects)	Outcome Measures	Grading	Conclusion
Van Tuijl et al.	2002	Review	Several	Very low	Reliability of MMT has not yet been tested. Contradictory statements about the sensitivity of MMT. Hand-held dynamometry is regarded as an ideal supplement to the MMT. It is also suitable to replace isokinetic dynamometry for practical reasons. This review gives a good overview of many available hand function tests, without recommending one over the others. For ADL testing, BI, MBI, FIM, QIF and SCIM are recommended.
Yavuz et al.	1998	Case Series (29)	AMS/FIM/QIF	Very low	FIM and QIF strongly correlate with AMS. The percent of recovery on AMS correlated to gain in QIF scores.

Table 2.2: Evidentiary table – upper extremity motor function

First Author	Year	Design (total no. of subjects)	Outcome Measures	Grading	Conclusion
Lim et al.	2005	Retrosp. Cohort (67)	VRI	Low	The VRI showed adequate face validity and sensitivity to injury severity measured by the AIS.
Lynch et al.	1998	Prosp. Cohort (30)	FRT	Moderate	The FRT can detect differences in level of lesion and shows high test-retest reliability.

Table 2.3: Evidentiary table – lower extremity motor function

First Author	Year	Design (total no. of subjects)	Outcome Measures	Grading	Conclusion
Harvey et al.	1998	Case Series (20)	Wheelchair Test	Very low	The Wheelchair Test shows a high inter-rater reliability. It is a reliable method to assess mobility of paraplegic patients.
Kilkens et al.	2004	Prosp. Cohort (74)	Wheelchair Circuit	Moderate	The Wheelchair Circuit is a valid and responsive tool to measure manual wheelchair mobility.
Kirby et al.	2002	Case Series (24)	WST	Very low	The WST is a practical, safe test and shows good reliability, excellent content validity, but fair construct and concurrent validity and moderate usefulness.
May et al.	2003	Case Series (20)	4FTRWS	Very low	The 4FTRWS are practical, safe and reliable and can be used for clinical evaluation of wheelchair seating.

Table 2.4: Evidentiary table – wheelchair

First Author	Year	Design (total no. of subjects)	Outcome Measures	Grading	Conclusion
Barbeau et al.	2007	RCT (70)	6MWT/50FWT	High	Fast subjects show a difference in walking speed between the 6MWT and the 50MWT after 12 months of rehabilitation. But in general the outcome measures of the 50FWT and the 6MWT do not reflect separable domains of mobility.
Curt et al.	1997	Prosp. Cohort (104)	AMS/SEP	Moderate	In an early state of acute SCI, AMS and SEP can help assessing the outcome of ambulatory capacity. In the 6 months after SCI, AMS increased significantly, whereas SEP recordings did not change.

First Author	Year	Design (total no. of subjects)	Outcome Measures	Grading	Conclusion
Ditunno et al.	2009	Review	Several	Very low	Measures of walking function such as walking speed, walking distance and the WISCI are valid and reliable tools recommended for use in clinical trials to determine effectiveness. The evolution of improved outcome measures of impaired walking function in SCI, based on continued gait research remains highly relevant to clinical investigation.
Ditunno et al.	2008b	Prosp. Cohort (150)	FIM/LEMS/WISCI	Moderate	The study supports the hierarchical ranking of the WISCI scale and the correlation of WISCI levels to impairment (LEMS) in a clinical setting of four nations.
Ditunno et al.	2007	RCT (146)	Several	High	After the first 6 months of rehabilitation, WISCI correlated well with LEMS, FIM, locomotor FIM, 50FWT and 6MWT. Correlations of change scores from baseline WISCI were significant for change scores of baseline LEMS and locomotor FIM. WISCI shows good concurrent and predictive validity. A combination of 50FWT, BBS, LEMS, locomotor FIM and WISCI is recommended for monitoring ambulatory function in clinical trials.
Ditunno et al.	2000	Construct study	FIM/WISCI	Very low	The WISCI shows good validity and reliability
Dobkin et al.	2007	RCT (145)	AMS/FIM/50FWT	High	Walking speed of over 0.6m/s correlated with LEMS near 40 or higher. Time after SCI is an important variable for entering patients into a trial with mobility-related outcome. All walking-related outcome measures increased in the 12 first weeks of rehabilitation.
Gorassini et al.	2009	Case Series (17)	EMG	Very low	Increases in the amount and decreases in the duration of EMG activity of specific muscles are associated with functional recovery of walking skills after treadmill training in subjects that are able to modify muscle activity patterns following incomplete spinal cord injury.

First Author	Year	Design (total no. of subjects)	Outcome Measures	Grading	Conclusion
Jackson et al.	2008	Experts' opinion	Several	Very low	A combination of the 10MWT and WISCI would provide the most valid measure of improvement in gait and ambulation in as much as objective changes of speed, and functional capacity allow for interval measurement. To provide the most comprehensive battery, however, it will be important to include a measure of endurance such as the 6MWT.
Kim et al.	2007	Prosp. Cohort (50)	WISCI	Moderate	Ambulatory speed was higher for self-selected WISCI compared to maximal WISCI. Walking at self-selected WISCI was also less energy demanding.
Kim et al.	2004	Case Series (22)	AMS/8MWT/6MWT	Very low	Strength of hip flexors, extensors and abductors correlated well with gait speed, 6MWT distance and ambulatory capacity.
Lam et al.	2008	Review	Several	Very low	Excellent tools are available for measuring functional ambulation capacity. Further work is required to develop and evaluate outcome measures to include environmental factors that contribute to the ability to achieve safe, functional ambulation in everyday settings.
Morganti et al.	2005	Retrosp. Cohort (284)	AMS/FIM/SCIM/WISCI	Low	WISCI shows a good concurrent validity compared to the BI, FIM, RMI and SCIM. Further refinement of the scale is recommended.
Norton et al.	2006	Case Series (12)	EMG/MEP/WISCI	Very low	Increases in higher-frequency EMG coherence in subjects with residual voluntary muscle strength and its parallel relation to changes in TMS-evoked responses provide further evidence that increases in corticospinal drive to muscles of the leg mediate improvements in locomotor function from treadmill training.
Opara et al.	2007	Review	AMS/FIM/SCIM/WISCI	Very low	The WISCI is the most detailed scale that is also the most sensitive to changes in the patient's walking ability compared to the other scales.

First Author	Year	Design (total no. of subjects)	Outcome Measures	Grading	Conclusion
Scivoletto et al.	2009	Review	Several	Very low	The DPR has prognostic value to walking recovery during spinal shock phase. Early SEP predict motor improvement and ambulation outcome. MEP can contribute in predicting the recovery of functional movements. The LEMS is also a prognostic tool for regaining ambulatory function.
Thomas et al.	2005	Case Series (8)	Several	Very low	The percentage increase in MEP was correlated to the degree of locomotor recovery as assessed by the WISCI score, the distance a subject could walk in 6 min, and the amplitude of the locomotor EMG activity.
van Hedel et al.	2009	Retrosp. Cohort (886)	SCIM/WISCI	Low	The wheelchair and walking items of the SCIM II show good validity and responsiveness. They are appropriate for evaluating the efficacy of new interventions on ambulatory function.
van Hedel	2009	Retrosp. Cohort (886)	10MWT/SCIM	Low	In subjects with spinal cord injury, the preferred walking speed can be used to estimate functional ambulation during daily life. The walking speed can distinguish between ambulation categories with high sensitivity and specificity.
van Hedel et al.	2008	Retrosp. Cohort (917)	Several	Very low	It is suggested that the 10MWT might be the best choice for assessing walking capacity in SCI subjects. Furthermore, the additional assessment of the dependence of the SCI subjects on walking aids or personal assistance is recommended.
van Hedel et al.	2007a	Retrosp. Cohort (51)	6MWT/10MWT	Low	Incomplete SCI subjects prefer to walk closer to their maximal walking speed compared to control subjects. Both preferred and maximal walking speeds assessed by the 10MWT well predicted the walking speed of the 6MWT. Therefore the use of the 10MWT is recommended.
van Hedel et al.	2006	Case Series (22)	AMS/6MWT/ 10MWT/WISCI	Very low	6MWT and 10MWT are more responsive compared to WISCI II. To monitor improvement in locomotor capacity, the use of timed walking tests is recommended.

First Author	Year	Design (total no. of subjects)	Outcome Measures	Grading	Conclusion
van Hedel et al.	2005b	Prosp. Cohort (75)	Several	Moderate	The TUG, 10MWT and 6MWT are valid and reliable measures for assessing walking function in patients with SCI.
van Middendorp et al.	2008	Retrosp. Cohort (273)	10MWT/TUG	Low	10MWT and TUG have a higher prognostic value for the recovery of walking compared to the AIS conversion outcome measure.
Wirz et al.	2006	Retrosp. Cohort (178)	LEMS/10MWT/WISCI	Very low	An improvement in locomotor function does not always reflect an increase in LEMS, and vice versa.
Wirz et al.	2005	Case Series (20)	Several	Very low	Changes in LEMS did not correlate with changes in overground walking speed. The WISCI may be less sensitive to changes in specific interventions. The 10MWT, the 6MWT, and the TUG test are more sensitive.

Table 2.5: Evidentiary table – ambulation

First Author	Year	Design (total no. of subjects)	Grading	Conclusion
Deng et al.	2004	Retrospective cohort (92)	Low	Immediate admission to SCI rehab group had improved BI, FIM scores and motor recovery compared to delayed admission group
Sumida et al.	2001	Retrospective cohort (123)	Low	Admission to SCI rehab within 2 weeks resulted in improved motor recovery rate and FIM scores compared to 2 weeks to 6 months group and greater than 6 months group.
Scivoletto et al.	2005	Retrospective cohort (150)	Low	Matched cohorts grouped as admission < 30 days, 30-60 days, >60 days. Early group had better BI improvements, without confounding improved motor recovery

Table 2.6: Evidentiary table – timing of rehabilitation

3 Functional walking after incomplete spinal cord injury – should the 10 Meter Walk Test be curvy?

Published in modified form in the journal *Archives of Physical Medicine and Rehabilitation*: Labruyère R, van Hedel JA. Curve Walking Is Not Better Than Straight Walking in Estimating Ambulation-Related Domains After Incomplete Spinal Cord Injury. Arch Phys Med Rehabil. 2012;93(5):796-801

3.1 Abstract

Objectives: (1) To determine the ability of the 10 Meter Walk Test (10MWT) to estimate the walking capacity after incomplete spinal cord injury (iSCI) in more complex conditions mimicking environmentally demanding situations. (2) To investigate whether the 10MWT could be modified to better predict community functioning.

Design: Case-control study.

Setting: Spinal cord injury center of a university hospital in Switzerland.

Participants: A convenience sample of 15 iSCI subjects (mean age 50 years, 40% women, neurologic level from C3 to L5, median time since injury 5 months) was compared to an age-matched control group (47% women).

Intervention: Not applicable.

Main Outcome Measures: We developed the Figure of Eight Test (FET) with six conditions to test the subjects' ability to adapt their gait to several circumstances. These conditions covered normal and maximal walking speed, constraint vision, obstacles, foamed soles and a dual task. Additionally, subjects were tested for lower extremity muscle strength, gait capacity (10MWT) and balance, independence and fear of falling.

Results: (1) Preferred straight-walking speed correlated with the different FET conditions in both groups; (2) if normalized to preferred straight-walking speed FET conditions showed significant differences between both groups and (3) if normalized to preferred curve-walking speed, these differences seemed to disappear. (4) The 10MWT appeared superior to the various conditions of the FET in estimating various other walking-related functions.

Conclusion: iSCI subjects seem to have difficulties with curve-walking compared to straight-walking. We therefore recommend the implementation of curve-walking into rehabilitation training programs. However, curve-walking did not provide any additional information with respect to estimating functional ambulation performance after an iSCI.

3.2 Introduction

Walking tests are routinely used in clinical settings, especially in neurology where regaining or improvement of walking function is often a key goal. Mobility is rated one of the most important activities of daily living for people with neurologic disorders (Chiou and Burnett, 1985). For example, after an incomplete spinal cord injury (iSCI), improvement of locomotor function is one of the primary aims (Ditunno et al., 2008a). Therefore, mobility measures are important for rehabilitation. In scientific environments sophisticated methods of motion analysis are often used, like motion capturing, electromyographic recording or pedobarography. However, these tools are not always suitable for clinical use. Therefore, more simple measures of walking function have been developed to measure mobility in a clinical setting. Well-investigated examples with good reliability and validity in neurologic populations are the 10 Meter Walk Test (10MWT, van Hedel et al., 2005b), the 2 Minute Walk Test (Rossier and Wade, 2001), the 6 Minute Walk Test (Harada et al., 1999), the Timed Up & Go Test (van Hedel et al., 2005b) and the revised Walking Index for SCI (WISCI II, Ditunno and Ditunno, 2001). These tests give an insight into the general walking capacity of the subjects.

The 10MWT has shown a high correlation with the other timed tests and a good correlation with WISCI II in iSCI subjects (van Hedel et al., 2005b). Therefore, several groups recommended the 10MWT and the WISCI II as best validated scales for measuring walking capacity in that population (Labruyère et al., 2010; Ditunno, 2010; Alexander et al., 2009; Jackson et al., 2008; Steeves et al., 2007). Improvement in lower extremity motor scores according to the ASIA (American Spinal Injury Association) International Standards (Marino et al., 2003) explained most of the variance in improvement in WISCI II, hence linking body structure with walking capacity (Ditunno, 2010). A recent European Multicenter Study database publication took the same line by relating improvement in ASIA Impairment Scale (AIS) grades with 10MWT and WISCI II (van Hedel and Dietz, 2009). It has been suggested that the concurrent use of the 10MWT together with the WISCI II is superior to either test alone (Labruyère et al., 2010; Jackson et al., 2008). Jackson et al. stated that this combination might also improve clinical significance as it could serve as a marker of the participant's ability to function in the community (Jackson et al., 2008).

However, the question has been raised whether walking speed as assessed in the clinic can be used to declare functional walking during daily life (van Hedel, 2009). Functional walking has been defined as 'the ability to walk, with or without the aid of appropriate assistive devices, safely and sufficiently to carry out mobility-related activities of daily living' (Lam et al., 2008). Thus, for an assessment of functional walking maybe more is needed than just indoor walking straight ahead for 10m on a leveled floor (Musselman et al., 2011). Factors like curbs and stairs (Musselman et al., 2007), curves (Hess et al., 2009; Guglielmetti et al., 2009), uneven ground (Musselman et al., 2007), limited vision (van Hedel et al., 2005a) or cognitive challenges (Hess et al., 2009; Lajoie et al., 1999) could limit ambulatory performance (as opposed to capacity, Lam et al., 2008). Daily life walking often involves this added complexity. A complex walking task may call for greater demands of physical and mental capacity, resulting in a drop in gait performance not seen for simple walking tasks (Hess et al., 2009).

Still, however, out of five community independence criteria, it appeared that iSCI subjects had the most difficulty with reaching the required velocity to safely cross an intersection (Lapointe et al., 2001). Thus, walking speed might provide information about the ambulation performance capabilities of iSCI subjects. Indeed, van

Hedel and Dietz tried to determine the capability of the 10MWT to estimate functional ambulation during daily life after iSCI (van Hedel and Dietz, 2009). They found that within the time-frame of rehabilitation (approximately up to 6 months) the 10MWT correlated poor ($r = 0.37$) to relatively well ($r = 0.85$) with the Spinal Cord Independence Measure (SCIM, Itzkovich et al., 2007) mobility items, depending on time after lesion and severity of neurologic impairment (van Hedel and Dietz, 2009). Hence, it seems that further work is required to include environmental factors that contribute to the ability of achieving safe, functional ambulation in everyday settings. Especially, since almost 30% of spinal cord injured subjects are functional walkers one year post-injury (Daverat et al., 1988).

Therefore, the aim of this study was to determine the ability of the 10MWT to estimate walking capacity in more complex conditions mimicking environmentally or physically demanding situations. Furthermore, we addressed the question whether several modifications of the 10MWT could result in an improved predictive capacity of community ambulation.

3.3 Methods

3.3.1 Subjects

Criteria for inclusion in the study were as follows: (1) AIS C or D, (2) being able to walk independently in the community with or without assistive devices. Subjects who had neurologic impairments in addition to their iSCI were excluded from the study. Prior to testing, written informed consent was obtained from every participant and the study was approved by the ethics committee of the Canton of Zurich, Switzerland.

Fifteen subjects with iSCI (6 women) were recruited. They were 50.4±15.0 years old (mean ± standard deviation), ranging between 20 and 70 years, they were 170.7±11.7cm tall and weighed 72.7±13.7kg. Median time since injury was 4.9 months (range: 1.1–154.8 months). Nine subjects were inpatients of our spinal cord injury center (time since lesion < 7 months), while 6 persons were outpatients (time since lesion > 1 year). Neurologic lesion levels ranged from cervical 3 to lumbar 5. Two subjects were classified as AIS C and the others as AIS D.

Fifteen subjects (7 women) with no neurological or musculoskeletal disorders participated as controls to determine normative values. They were 50.3±14.5 years old (range: 23-68), 173.2±8.7cm tall and they weighed 74.1±12.1kg. The control group was frequency matched to the iSCI group, therefore both groups were equal for age ($p=0.99$), height ($p=0.52$) and weight ($p=0.77$).

3.3.2 Measurement of functional walking

To test the subjects' ability to adapt their gait to several circumstances, we developed the Figure of Eight Test (FET) with different conditions. The figure of eight had a length of 10m to allow comparisons with the 10MWT. It consisted of 2 adjacent circles with a radius of each 160cm (Figure 3.1). Path width was 80cm to ensure that the test could also be done with a walker. The path that had to be followed was marked with tape and delimited with cones. All subjects started and ended their walking at least 1.5m outside the figure of eight to minimize acceleration and deceleration effects. The outcome measure was time needed for one lap for every condition. The stopwatch was started as soon as the first foot crossed the dashed midline (Figure 3.1) and it was stopped as the first foot crossed the dashed midline again after one lap. All trials were recorded on video to control times offline. The results of all walking tests were converted to walking speed (m/s).

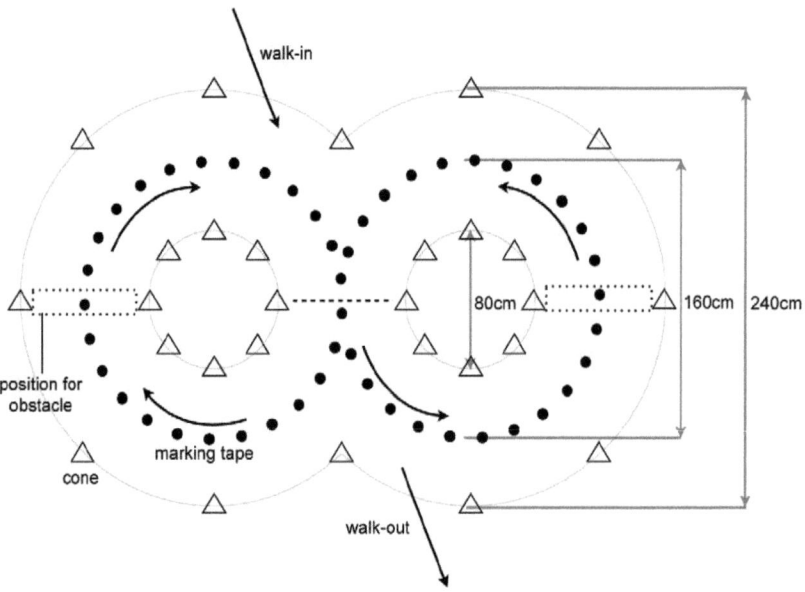

Figure 3.1: Schematic drawing of the figure of eight test. Round arrows indicate walking direction.

The FET consisted of 6 different conditions mimicking several specific demands of functional walking:

- Normal FET (FET normal): This provided insight in difficulties with turning – which might increase demands for balance – in contrast to the straight-walking 10MWT.
- Maximal FET (FET maximal): FET normal at maximal safe walking speed.
- Limited vision FET (FET vision): Subjects wore glasses simulating cataract (blurred view, 10% of normal vision). This emphasized dependence on vision.
- Obstacle FET (FET obstacle): Two obstacles (one in each curve, Figure 3.1) with a width of 60cm, height of 10cm and a depth of 7cm had to be overstepped. The height of the obstacle corresponded to an average curb in Switzerland.
- Foam-soles FET (FET foam): Subjects wore foamed soles under their shoes. This emphasized dependence on the proprioceptive system.
- Dual task FET (FET dual): During walking, a number of questions had to be answered as quickly as possible. This provided information about the amount of "automaticity" of walking, i.e. the attentional demand required for walking.

Except for FET maximal, subjects were directed to walk at self-selected speed corresponding to their preferred comfortable walking speed in everyday life. Instructions were as follows: "Walk into the figure of eight starting in a counterclockwise direction at a comfortable speed / as fast as you can and begin when I say 'go'. Follow the black dots". Subjects who had difficulties with walking were accompanied by an assisting person to minimize the risk of a fall. The conditions were applied in a randomized order and between the conditions there was a break of at least 30s. All subjects performed a test trial (FET normal) to familiarize with the test. To analyze the influence of curves on walking speed the FET conditions were normalized to preferred straight-walking speed and to analyze the influence of the additional tasks on walking speed the FET conditions were normalized to FET normal.

3.3.3 Additional measurements

For iSCI subjects, etiology and level of lesion, AIS, time since SCI and medication was documented. To quantify mobility, the indoors and outdoors mobility part of the latest version of the SCIM (herein after referred to as 'SCIM mobility', from *0 = no mobility* to *30 = normal mobility*) was assessed in all subjects together with the WISCI II (from *0 = unable to walk* to *20 = able to walk without assistive devices*). Muscle strength of the legs was examined with the lower extremity motor score (LEMS, from *0 = complete paralysis* to *50 = normal strength*, Marino et al., 2003). The international version of the Falls Efficacy Scale (FES, from *16 = not at all concerned* to *64 = very concerned,* Yardley et al., 2005) was applied to quantify fear of falling in order to account for a psychological aspect of functional walking. The 10MWT was used to assess gait capacity. It was performed at preferred and maximum speed. Recorded was the time required to walk the intermediate 10m of a 14m walkway. As in the FET this was done to minimize acceleration and deceleration effects. To assess static balance under different conditions we applied the Sensory Organization Test (SOT, from *6 = minimal sway in all conditions* to *24 = fall in all conditions,* Anacker et al., 1992). This test consisted of quiet standing for 30s on a firm and a compliant support surface during three visual conditions (eyes open, eyes closed and visual stabilization using a helmet dome). This amounted to 6 different conditions each of which was scored from *1 = minimal sway* to *4 = fall*. These scores were then summed up to one final score (a more detailed description on the SOT has been published earlier, Shumway-Cook and Horak, 1986). This test was chosen, because all different SOT conditions require a differentiated dependence on the visual, vestibular and somatosensory system that are all directly linked with walking function (Lord et al., 1991).

This assessment battery was used to address the complex spectrum of walking function, physiologically as well as psychologically.

3.3.4 Statistical analysis

The relationship between the different tests was investigated using correlation analyses and linear regression. Correlations were quantified with Pearson's rank correlation coefficients (r) for normally distributed data and with Spearman's Rho (ρ) for ordinal data. Differences between the iSCI group and controls were quantified with the Independent Samples T Test (normally distributed data) and with the Mann-Whitney U Test (not normally distributed data). Normality of distribution was tested with the Shapiro-Wilk Test. To compare the strength of the 10MWT and FET variables in predicting measures of function, we used simple linear regression analyses to explain the variability of SCIM mobility, LEMS, FES, WISCI II and SOT. All the statistics were done using PASW Statistics 17 (IBM Corporation, New York, USA).

3.4 Results

There were significant differences for all outcome measures between controls and iSCI subjects (Table 3.1). Controls as well as iSCI subjects were able to safely perform all 6 FET conditions. Correlations with age were not found, except with the maximal 10MWT and maximal FET in controls (r=-0.61, p=0.02; r=-0.53, p=0.04). Correlations between different FET conditions ranged from r=-0.16 (FET maximal vs. FET visual) to r=0.90 (FET normal vs. FET obstacle) for controls and from ρ=0.72 (FET visual vs. FET obstacle) to ρ=0.94 (FET normal vs. FET dual) for patients.

If figure of eight walking speeds were normalized to preferred straight-walking speed (assessed with the 10MWT), there were significant differences for all but one condition between controls and iSCI subjects (Table 3.2). However, if figure of eight walking speeds were normalized to preferred curve-walking speed (assessed with the FET normal), only one condition revealed significant differences between controls and iSCI subjects (Table 3.2). In Table 3.3 correlations between 10MWT and FET conditions are depicted for both groups. In iSCI subjects, preferred straight-walking speed correlated better with measures of function compared to preferred curve-walking speed (Table 3.4).

Linear regression models showed that in iSCI subjects variation in normal 10MWT explained a major part of the variation of the different FET conditions (adjusted R^2=91% for FET normal, 91% for FET maximal, 92% for FET visual, 87% for FET obstacle, 85% for FET foam and 82% for FET dual). Figure 3.2 shows that the variation in preferred 10MWT explained in most cases a larger amount of variation of the outcome measures of function compared to the different FET conditions. The explained variance values of the FET maximal behaved similar to and did not significantly differ from those of the FET normal. Therefore, they were not depicted in Figure 3.2.

	Controls	iSCI subjects	P-values
Normal 10MWT [m/s]	1.46 ± 0.21	0.93 ± 0.29	< 0.001
Maximal 10MWT [m/s]	2.22 ± 0.34	1.23 ± 0.44	< 0.001
10MWT normal/maximal ratio [%]	67.1 ± 13.0	77.8 ± 11.3	0.072
FET normal [m/s]	1.29 ± 0.19	0.75 ± 0.29	< 0.001
FET maximal [m/s]	1.88 ± 0.38	0.97 ± 0.39	< 0.001
FET visual [m/s]	1.30 ± 0.16	0.73 ± 0.36	< 0.001
FET obstacle [m/s]	1.28 ± 0.15	0.72 ± 0.37	0.001
FET foam [m/s]	1.22 ± 0.21	0.62 ± 0.36	< 0.001
FET dual [m/s]	1.17 ± 0.21	0.71 ± 0.31	< 0.001
FET normal/maximal ratio [%]	70.2 ± 13.6	77.8 ± 7.7	0.042
LEMS	50.0 ± 0.0	43.4 ± 7.2	< 0.001
FES	16.9 ± 1.6	24.2 ± 7.0	< 0.001
SCIM mobility	30.0 ± 0.0	23.1 ± 5.0	< 0.001
WISCI II	20.0 ± 0.0	16.9 ± 2.8	0.001
SOT sum	8.6 ± 1.0	14.4 ± 4.5	< 0.001

Table 3.1: Averages and standard deviations of results for patients and controls. P-values for differences between groups, grey colored fields indicate non-parametric testing; iSCI = incomplete spinal cord injury; 10MWT = 10 Meter Walk Test, FET = Figure of Eight Test,

LEMS = lower extremity motor score, FES = Falls Efficacy Scale, SCIM = Spinal Cord Independence Measure, WISCI = Walking Index for Spinal Cord Injury, SOT = Sensory Organization Test.

Normalized to	Normal 10MWT			Normal FET		
	Controls	iSCI subjects	P-values	Controls	iSCI subjects	P-values
FET normal	88.1 ± 7.7	79.4 ± 8.1	0.005	n.a.	n.a	n.a.
FET maximal	130.9 ± 31.8	102.9 ± 13.7	0.008	148.6 ± 35.0	129.7 ± 12.9	0.148
FET visual	90.2 ± 11.9	75.9 ± 13.2	0.005	102.2 ± 9.5	95.6 ± 12.9	0.122
FET obstacle	88.3 ± 9.7	72.2 ± 16.6	0.003	100.2 ± 6.9	90.8 ± 17.3	0.062
FET foam	82.8 ± 7.4	63.6 ± 16.8	<0.001	94.3 ± 8.2	79.7 ± 15.9	0.004
FET dual	80.2 ± 8.9	75.3 ± 12.7	0.226	91.3 ± 10.0	94.6 ± 10.2	0.381

Table 3.2: Averages and standard deviations of results of the FET normalized to 10MWT normal and FET normal (in %). P-values for differences between groups, grey colored fields indicate non-parametric testing; iSCI = incomplete spinal cord injury; 10MWT = 10 Meter Walk Test, FET = Figure of Eight Test.

		FET normal	FET maximal	FET visual	FET obstacle	FET foam	FET dual
Controls	Normal 10MWT	0.83 ***	0.09	0.55 *	0.73 **	0.91 ***	0.75 **
	Maximal 10MWT	0.09	0.58 *	0.05	0.19	0.31	0.26
iSCI subjects	Normal 10MWT	0.89 ***	0.72 **	0.90 ***	0.63 *	0.84 ***	0.90 ***
	Maximal 10MWT	0.81 ***	0.85 ***	0.75 **	0.65 *	0.89 ***	0.84 ***

Table 3.3: Correlations between straight-walking and curve-walking tests. * $p \leq 0.05$, ** $p \leq 0.01$ and *** $p \leq 0.001$ for significance of correlations; Grey colored fields indicate Spearman correlations;

10MWT = 10 Meter Walk Test, FET = Figure of Eight Test, iSCI = incomplete spinal cord injury.

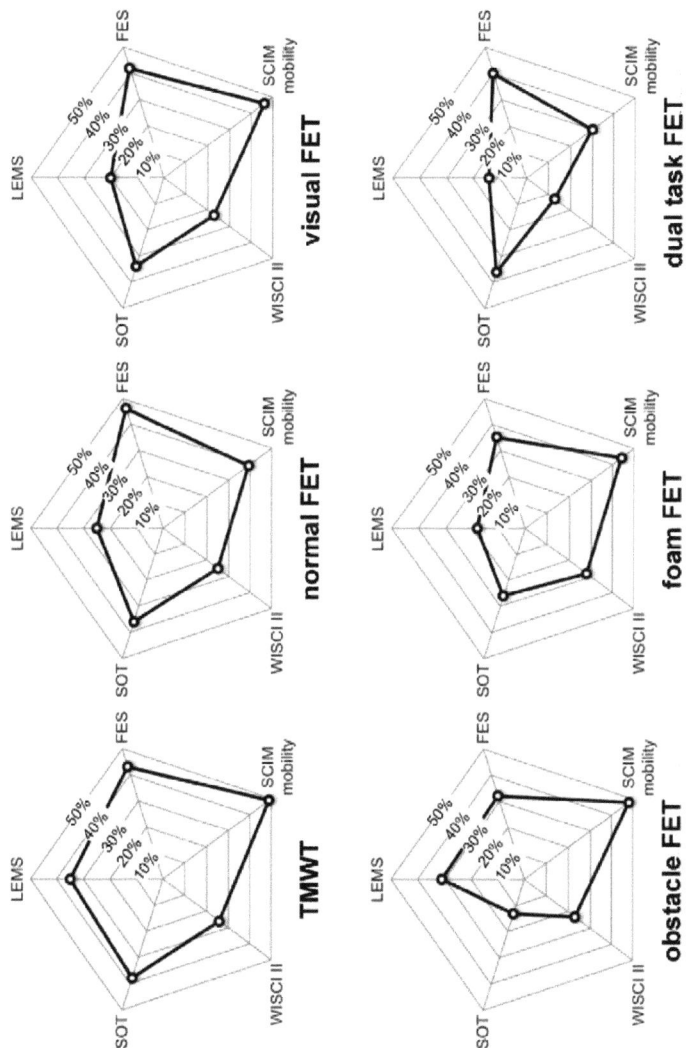

Figure 3.2: Visualization of the linear regression analyses in incomplete spinal cord injured subjects. Spider diagrams show the

amount of explained variation of the measures of function by the different walk tests. TMWT = 10 Meter Walk Test, FET = Figure of Eight Test, LEMS = lower extremity motor score, FES = Falls Efficacy Scale, SCIM = Spinal Cord Independence Measure, WISCI = Walking Index for Spinal Cord Injury, SOT = Sensory Organization Test.

	LEMS	FES	SCIM mobility	WISCI	SOT
Normal 10MWT	0.66 **	- 0.62 *	0.67 **	0.5	- 0.75 **
Normal FET	0.59 *	- 0.82 ***	0.52 *	0.46	- 0.67 **

Table 3.4: Correlations between measures of function and 10MWT normal and FET normal in incomplete spinal cord injured subjects. * $p \leq 0.05$, ** $p \leq 0.01$ and *** $p \leq 0.001$ for significance of correlations; Grey colored fields indicate Spearman correlations; 10MWT = 10 Meter Walk Test, FET = Figure of Eight Test, LEMS = lower extremity motor score, FES = Falls Efficacy Scale, SCIM = Spinal Cord Independence Measure, WISCI = Walking Index for Spinal Cord Injury, SOT = Sensory Organization Test.

3.5 Discussion

Our purpose of this study was to investigate the ability of the 10MWT to estimate walking capacity in more complex conditions mimicking environmentally or physically demanding situations. A secondary aim was to investigate whether the 10MWT could be improved by modifying several features in such a way that it might predict community functioning to a higher extent.

The main findings were the following: (1) In general, preferred straight-walking speed correlated well with the different conditions of the FET in controls as well as iSCI subjects; (2) if normalized to preferred straight-walking speed FET conditions showed significant differences between controls and iSCI subjects and (3) if normalized to preferred curve-walking speed, these differences seemed to disappear. (4) The 10MWT appeared superior compared to the various conditions of the FET in estimating various other walking-related functions and performance.

3.5.1 Ambulatory capacity versus performance

In iSCI subjects the preferred and maximal 10MWT correlated moderately to well with our walking capacity measures (FET) that reflected more complex conditions mimicking environmental or physical demanding conditions. This was only partially the case in healthy subjects, either due to a lesser statistical spread of data points or due to the simplicity of the tasks. Nevertheless, correlations between preferred straight-walking speed and preferred curve-walking speed in healthy subjects were higher compared to those of a recent study (Guglielmetti et al., 2009). Since the FET conditions were thought to mimic some specific demands of functional walking, we hypothesized that they also might be superior over the 10MWT in explaining the variation in measures of daily life ambulation. We therefore thought it might be a suitable measure of ambulatory performance. However, linear regression models showed that this was not the case and that the preferred 10MWT often even explained more of the variation of the performed measures of function compared to the different FET conditions. Apparently, curves and additional tasks did not add any information about ambulatory performance compared to straight walking.

3.5.2 Influence of curves on walking speed

Apparently iSCI subjects did not seem to have problems with additional tasks that had to be accomplished in the different FET conditions, as almost no significant group differences were found when FET results were normalized to preferred curve-walking speed. It rather seems difficult for them to walk curves in the figure of eight, as the normalized (for preferred straight-walking speed) values differed between the groups. Curve-walking indeed is more difficult than straight-walking. According to a recent paper of Guglielmetti et al. there are several differences between straight- and curve-walking, for example a change in the spatiotemporal pattern of muscle activation. Furthermore, there are differences for the inner and outer foot, such as different swing velocities, angles in foot placement, stance phase durations and ground reaction forces. Finally, the mediolateral displacement of body center of mass toward the supporting leg is shifted inwards, to create the centripetal force that keeps the body moving along the circular path (Guglielmetti et al., 2009).

Indeed, this latter factor indicates that the demands are higher for curve-walking compared to straight-walking not only with respect to kinetics and kinematics but also to balance and even attention (Guglielmetti et al., 2009; Lapointe et al., 2001). Such gait adaptations for curved paths might especially be difficult for iSCI subjects, because gait patterns and locomotion in general are significantly altered due to decreased strength, proprioception, use of bracing, and spasticity (Jackson et al., 2008). In our study, the tight curve in the figure of eight (extrinsic curvature of 0.63/m) might have increased the required demands even more. To our knowledge, this study shows for the first time that walking along a curve seems to be a remarkably difficult task for iSCI subjects and at present, current gait assessments for this population do not deliberately account for the motor skills necessary for curve-walking (the Timed Up & Go Test and the 6 Minute Walk Test usually cover turns rather than curves).

3.5.3 Can the 10MWT be improved by making it curved?

Our results and the last two paragraphs indicate that curve-walking might be an underestimated task of activities of daily living after iSCI. From a clinical point of view it therefore makes sense to approach this actively during rehabilitation and specifically practice curve-walking in therapy. However, our analyses suggest no need for an additional outcome measure that includes active curve-walking in iSCI subjects, since the preferred 10MWT explains variability in measures of function better compared to the FET conditions. Our results also show that the preferred 10MWT seems to be superior over the maximal 10MWT in explaining variability of functional measures, as opposed to an earlier suggestion (van Hedel et al., 2007a). Nevertheless it makes sense to assess the maximal 10MWT, since it measures a different domain of walking and it outweighs the ceiling effect of the preferred 10MWT (Jackson et al., 2008).

3.5.4 Limitations of the study

The sample of subjects assessed in the current study was relatively small, which might limit the generalizability of our results. Nevertheless, the findings appear robust, as for example the normal/maximal straight-walking speed ratios from this study (controls: ratio=67%; iSCI subjects: ratio=78%) were well comparable to those reported in a previous study (van Hedel et al., 2007a) that evaluated 31 control subjects (ratio=59%) and 31 iSCI subjects (ratio=74%). In the FET conditions investigators had to walk closely behind the iSCI subjects for safety reasons, which may have influenced the pacing of the subjects. Furthermore, iSCI subjects already walked at a quite fair speed, about two-thirds of normal speed. Therefore, further studies might investigate the influence of walking curves on the gait pattern of iSCI subjects with poorer ambulatory capacity.

3.6 Conclusion

Our study showed that iSCI subjects have some difficulties with curve-walking compared to straight-walking and therefore we recommend the specific implementation of curve-walking into rehabilitation training programs. However, compared to the standard 10MWT, curve-walking did not provide any additional information with respect to estimating functional ambulation performance after an iSCI.

3.7 Acknowledgement

We sincerely thank the subjects for their participation and Marion Zimmerli for her help in performing the tests. This study was granted by the International Spinal Research Trust (Clinical Initiative Stage 2, London, Great Britain) and the EMDO Foundation (Zurich, Switzerland). We further acknowledge the Neuroscience Center Zurich (ZNZ) and the Rehabilitation Initiative and Technology Platform Zurich (RITZ).

4 Instrument validity and reliability of a choice response time test for incomplete spinal cord injured subjects: relationship with function

Published in the journal *Archives of Physical Medicine and Rehabilitation*: Labruyère R, van Hedel JA. Instrument validity and reliability of a choice response time test for incomplete spinal cord injured subjects: relationship with function. Arch Phys Med Rehabil. 2011;92(9):1443-9.

4.1 Abstract

Objectives: To investigate instrument validity and reliability of a choice response time (CRT) test for the lower extremities in incomplete spinal cord injured (iSCI) subjects. CRT in iSCI subjects is hypothesized to be increased due to, for example, muscle weakness or increased corticospinal conduction velocity.

Design: Case-control study for assessing instrument validity and reliability.

Setting: SCI center of a university hospital in Switzerland

Participants: Instrument validity was assessed by comparing CRTs of 28 patients with iSCI (mean age 51 years, 57% men, neurologic level from C3 to L5, median time since injury 148 days) with those of age matched controls (50% men). Reliability was determined in a subgroup of 9 iSCI subjects and 13 controls.

Intervention: Not applicable.

Main Outcome Measures: Choice response times of the lower extremity were assessed and divided into reaction and movement times. Additionally, iSCI subjects were tested for lower extremity muscle strength, gait capacity and mobility, independence, history of falls and fear of falling.

Results: CRTs of the control group (517±71ms, mean ± standard deviation) were significantly faster compared to those of the iSCI group (743±177ms; p<0.001). Retest reliability was high in controls (ICC>0.98) and iSCI subjects (ICC>0.93). In iSCI subjects there were moderate to good correlations between CRT and several functional outcome measures, but not with the reported number of falls.

Conclusion: Lower extremity CRT testing appears reliable in healthy as well as ambulating iSCI subjects.

4.2 Introduction

International numbers on the incidence of spinal cord injury (SCI) vary between 10 to 83 persons per million every year (Wyndaele and Wyndaele, 2006). Approximately 50% of these patients suffer from a sensory-motor incomplete lesion, that is, sensory and/or motor function is partially preserved below the level of lesion (Wyndaele and Wyndaele, 2006; National Spinal Cord Injury Statistical Center Facts&Figures, 2010). One of the primary goals of rehabilitating incomplete SCI (iSCI) patients is regaining ambulatory function (Anderson, 2004). Statistically, 50% to 95% of iSCI subjects succeed in doing so (Consortium for Spinal Cord Medicine, 2000; Burns et al., 1997). However, ambulation seldom becomes normative and these individuals tend to walk slower, depend on walking aids (van Hedel et al., 2008) and are prone to falling (Wirz et al., 2009; Brotherton et al., 2007). Underlying causes for this can be spasticity or an impairment of balance, strength or proprioception (Scivoletto et al., 2008). Also a prolongation of response times of the lower extremities might affect walking performance (Lord and Fitzpatrick, 2001; Woolley et al., 1997; Lord and Clark, 1996; Patla et al., 1993), but has received little attention in iSCI patients.

In healthy subjects, response times are subject to age-related changes; already before 1900, simple response times were found to be significantly slower in aged subjects (Ruger and Stoessiger, 1927), and this finding has been confirmed repeatedly, also for choice response time (CRT) tasks (for references, see Spirduso, 1975; Welford, 1977). Delayed response times can lead to walking-related issues (Lord and Fitzpatrick, 2001; Patla et al., 1993), and this might especially affect iSCI subjects. However, it remains unclear, whether response times are really increased in iSCI subjects. Indeed, since the conduction time of the corticospinal tract is often prolonged after iSCI (Diehl et al., 2006; Calancie et al., 1999), and the strength of partially paralyzed muscles (van Hedel et al., 2010) is reduced, CRT is hypothesized to be affected.

In SCI rehabilitation there are clinical assessments for sensory and motor function (Labruyère et al., 2010; Marino et al., 2003), independence of activities of daily living (Itzkovich et al., 2007), walking ability (van Hedel and Dietz, 2009; Ditunno et al., 2008b) and balance (Wirz et al., 2009; Boswell-Ruys et al., 2009; Datta et al., 2009). However, there is no validated test to assess response time, although a timely correct foot placement plays an important role in quickly adjusting the locomotor pattern for safe locomotion (Chen et al., 1994). Unlike in other neurologic conditions like Huntington, multiple sclerosis, Parkinson's disease or stroke (Solomon et al., 2008; Marcotte et al., 2008; Mazzucchi et al., 1993; Melzer et al., 2009), there appears to be only 1 study that examined response time after iSCI by investigating the braking response times in a driving simulator equipped with hand-driven levers (Peters, 2001). We therefore developed a device for the lower extremities to examine CRT in iSCI subjects. The aims of this study were (i) to validate the CRT device for its use in iSCI subjects, (ii) to compare the response times of iSCI subjects with functional measures, and (iii) to determine the retest reliability.

4.3 Methods

4.3.1 Subjects

Twenty-eight subjects (14 women) with no neurologic or musculoskeletal conditions participated as controls to determine normative values. They were on average 51.4±11.2 years old (mean ± standard deviation) and 172.0±9.3cm tall.

Furthermore, 28 iSCI subjects participated (12 women). The subjects were 51.1±14.2 years old and 169.9±11.2cm tall. Median time since injury was 148 days (range: 24 days – 31.9 years). Neurologic lesion levels ranged from cervical 3 to lumbar 5. The median Walking Index for Spinal Cord Injury (WISCI) was 16 (ambulating with two crutches, no braces and no physical assistance) and varied between 9 (ambulating with walker, with braces, but no physical assistance) and 20 (ambulating with no devices, no braces and no physical assistance). One subject was classified as ASIA Impairment Scale (AIS, Marino et al., 2003) C (Neurologic level: lumbar 3; lower extremity motor score [LEMS]: 25; and, WISCI: 16, i.e. ambulating with two crutches) and the others were AIS D. Seventeen were inpatients (time since lesion < 1 year) of our SCI center, while 11 subjects were outpatients (time since lesion > 1 year).

The exclusion criteria were: Not being able to walk, impaired vision not correctable with glasses or contact lenses and inability to understand simple instructions. Prior to testing, written informed consent was obtained from every participant and the study was approved by the ethics committee of the Canton of Zurich, Switzerland.

4.3.2 Device

The Reaction and Execution Test (RET) device (Figure 4.1) consists of a platform (57cm × 57cm × 3.5cm) containing 6 touch-sensors with a diameter of 1cm. Five target buttons are positioned in a semicircle 15cm from the tip of the starting position of the foot. In the starting position, 1 button is located under the heel of the foot. Next to each target button there is a corresponding blue light emitting diode (LED). These LEDs flash up pseudo-randomly in 6 randomized differing blocks of each 5 stimuli (30 stimuli in total) to ensure an even distribution over all target buttons. The interstimulus interval is between 1.2 and 5.2s. The heel button serves to divide the response time into reaction time, the time from flashing of the

LED till release of the heel button, and movement time, the time from release of the heel button till activation of the target button (analog to Spirduso, 1975). To avoid a sliding movement away from the heel button, rough-surfaced tape ensured proper foot lifting. Switches under every button recorded the time of stepping events within 1ms accuracy.

4.3.3 Data collection
In the control group, the RET was performed in a sitting position and in 15 subjects additionally also in a standing position. As seen in pretests it appeared difficult for some iSCI subjects to perform the RET in a sitting position, especially for those with weak knee and hip flexor muscle strength, therefore all iSCI subjects performed the RET in a standing position. The subjects were positioned between parallel bars and instructed to hold onto them during the test to prevent possible falls and to diminish the influence of corrective postural behavior.

To investigate test-retest reliability, 9 iSCI and 13 control subjects were asked to repeat the RET 1 day to 6 weeks after their first test at the same daytime and under similar circumstances.

4.3.4 Measuring response time
The RET was performed with one foot at a time (the test was done for both feet), the other foot was comfortably placed in the lower corner of the platform. When a LED flashed up, the foot had to be positioned as quickly as possible on the associated target button.

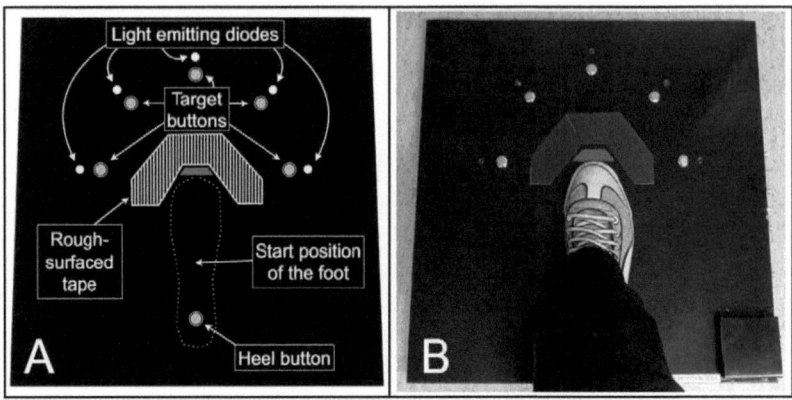

Figure 4.1: A: Schematic drawing of the Reaction and Execution Test device, B: Actual device with the foot in starting position.

After this target button was pressed, the LED turned off and the subject moved the foot back to the starting position at a self-selected speed. As soon as the heel was placed back on the heel button, a new trial started. The 3 quickest reaction and movement time trials per target button were averaged for each foot. These position-dependent values were then averaged to one reaction and one movement time for each foot separately and were then used for further analysis. Reaction times quicker than 100ms were considered false starts and not included in the analysis, just like each failed attempt, in which the target button was missed in the first attempt. All subjects performed at least 5 practice trials to familiarize with the task. Device control software was written in LabVIEW 8.2.1 (National Instruments Corporation, Austin, Texas, USA). The control software caused minimal but variable delays (0–5ms) in the recorded reaction and movement times. However, as we selected the 3 quickest reaction and movement times, we assumed that potential inaccuracies were kept to a minimum.

4.3.5 Additional measurements

For all subjects, general characteristics and foot dominance (i.e. "which foot is used to kick a ball?", Gabbard and Hart, 1996) were obtained by questionnaire. For iSCI subjects, etiology and level of lesion, AIS, time since SCI and medication was documented. Muscle strength of their lower extremities was examined with the LEMS (Marino et al., 2003). The international version of the Falls Efficacy Scale (FES-I, Yardley et al., 2005) was applied to quantify fear of falling and subjects were asked for their fall history over 1 month (Wirz et al., 2009) and 1 year retrospectively. Furthermore, to quantify gait capacity and mobility of the iSCI subjects, the mobility part of the latest Spinal Cord Independence Measure (SCIM, Itzkovich et al., 2007) was assessed together with the revised Walking Index for Spinal Cord Injury (WISCI, Ditunno and Ditunno, 2001) and the 10 Meter Walk Test (10MWT, van Hedel and Dietz, 2009). The 10MWT was performed at preferred and maximum speed. Recorded was the time required to walk the intermediate 10m of a 14m walkway. This was done to minimize acceleration and deceleration effects (see also van Hedel et al., 2007a).

4.3.6 Statistical Analysis

Our CRT measurements did not show a positively skewed distribution, as one would expect from literature (Miller et al., 1988), we therefore applied parametric testing (intra-group comparisons:

Paired Samples T Test; inter-group comparisons: Independent Samples T Test). Correlations were quantified with Pearson's rank correlation coefficients (r) for normally distributed data and with Spearman's Rho (ρ) for ordinal data. We quantified test-retest reliability using intraclass correlation coefficients (ICC), for which a 2 factor mixed effects model (type consistency) was performed, and the smallest real difference (SRD) was calculated and the number of subjects reaching the SRD-criterion were indicated as suggested in a previous study (Schuck and Zwingmann, 2003). Intra-individual strength differences between the legs in iSCI subjects were compared with a Wilcoxon Signed Rank test. For the age dependency of CRT in iSCI subjects, we performed a partial correlation analysis. All the statistics were done using PASW Statistics 17 (IBM Corporation, New York, USA).

4.4 Results

4.4.1 Control subjects

The average CRT for controls was 517±71ms. It comprised of reaction time (292±29ms) and movement time (225±48ms). The distribution of the data is depicted in Figure 4.2. Twenty-three subjects were right-footed, 2 were left-footed and 3 subjects had no preference. There was no significant difference between the dominant and the non-dominant foot for reaction time (293±31 vs. 294±31ms, p=0.83), as opposed to movement time (220±52 vs. 234±52ms, p=0.035). Sex-specific differences were not found, neither for reaction time (men: 291±31ms vs. women: 293±28ms, p=0.81), nor for movement time (217±56 vs. 233±40ms, p=0.39).

There was a moderate to strong relationship between age and CRT (Figure 4.3). In controls, there was no difference between CRTs in sitting vs. standing position (429±50 vs. 421±45ms, p=0.29, n=15).

4.4.2 iSCI subjects

The average CRT for iSCI subjects was 743±177ms and this was significantly slower compared to the controls (p<0.001). Also the average reaction time (381±65ms, p<0.001) and movement time (362±124ms, p<0.001) were slower (Figure 4.2). Twenty of the subjects were right-footed, 7 left-footed and 1 subject reported no preference. There was no significant difference between the dominant and the non-dominant foot for reaction time (376±73 vs. 375±69ms, p=0.92) nor for movement time (365±144 vs. 335±94ms, p=0.18). There was a significant difference between the stronger and the weaker leg (measured with LEMS for 19 patients with strength asymmetry, strong: 21.7±3.6 vs. weak: 17.5±5.9, p<0.001); this however did not influence reaction time (403±93 vs. 385±80 ms, p=0.44), as opposed to movement time (361±96 vs. 443±163 ms, p=0.006). Similar to the controls, sex-specific differences were not found, neither for reaction time (men: 379±72ms vs. women: 382±58ms, p=0.92) nor movement time (360±122 vs. 366±131ms, p=0.90). However, in contrast to the controls, there was no significant correlation between age and CRT (Figure 4.4). To exclude that the neurologic impairment might have masked a potential age effect on CRT, a partial correlation analysis was performed. The partial correlation coefficient of the 1st order for age and CRT of iSCI subjects did not change significantly after

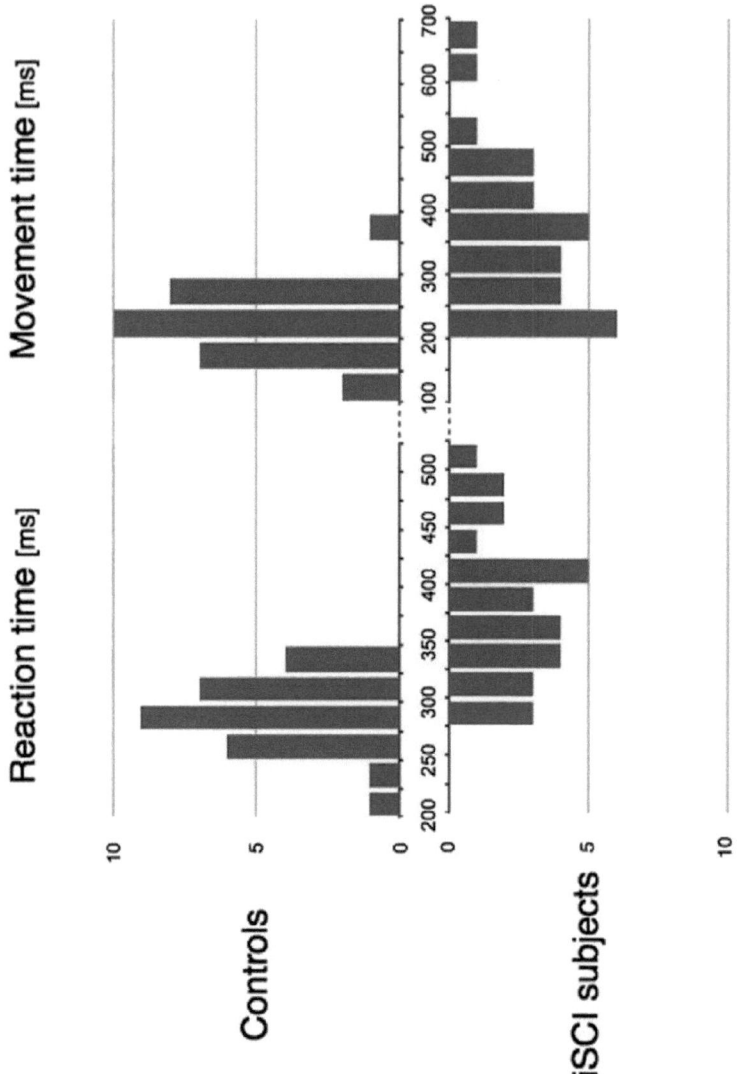

Figure 4.2: Distribution of reaction and movement times for controls and incomplete spinal cord injured subjects (iSCI) in the form of histograms.

controlling for LEMS (Bivariate correlation: -0.16, p=0.42; Partial correlation: 0.18, p=0.38).

Results of the additional measurement in iSCI subjects can be found in Table 4.1. With respect to the functional status of the iSCI patients, a moderate correlation between CRT and maximal walking speed (obtained from the 10MWT) was observed (Figure 4.4). However, when CRT was divided into reaction and movement times, correlations with maximal walking speed disappeared (r=-0.05, p=0.82 and r=-0.20, p=0.32). The same was true for moderate correlations between CRT and the WISCI, the mobility part of the SCIM and the FES-I (Figure 4.4). If split up into reaction and movement time, correlation coefficients were as follows: WISCI: r=-0.42, p=0.83 and r=-0.25, p=0.21; SCIM mobility part: r=-0.25, p=0.20 and r=-0.27, p=0.16; FES-I: r=0.30, p=0.14 and r=0.37, p=0.07. Also comparisons between CRT and its own sub-domains did not reveal significant correlations (reaction time: r=0.06, p=0.75, movement time: r=0.12, p=0.56). There was no significant association between the number of reported falls and CRT. This holds true for the fall history over 1 month as well as over 1 year (Figure 4.4).

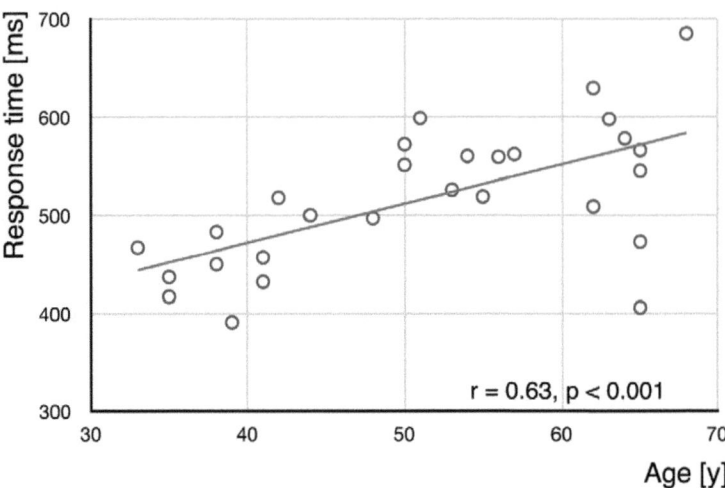

Figure 4.3: Correlation between age and choice response time in controls.

Measures	Mean ± SD	Range
Lower extremity motor score	42 ± 8	21 - 50
SCIM - mobility part	21 ± 7	8 - 30
Revised Walking Index for Spinal Cord Injury	16 ± 3	9 - 20
Preferred walking speed (m/s)	0.75 ± 0.42	0.08 - 1.67
Maximal walking speed (m/s)	0.86 ± 0.55	0.08 - 2.22
Falls Efficacy Scale - International Version	25 ± 11	16 - 53
Falls last month	0.3 ± 1.0	0 - 5
Falls last year	1.2 ± 2.2	0 - 10

Table 4.1: Mean results of several functional and fall-related measures in the incomplete spinal cord injured subjects. Abbreviations: SD = standard deviation; SCIM = Spinal Cord Independence Measure.

4.4.3 Reliability

The retest was performed on average 15±18 days (range: 1–56 days) after the first test. The test-retest reliability of the RET appeared excellent, as the ICC in controls was 0.987 with a 95% CI from 0.958–0.996. The mean between-day variation for the RET was 7±22ms. The SRD was 44ms and 92% (12 out of 13 controls) reached the SRD-criterion. The ICC for iSCI subjects was 0.930 with a 95% CI from 0.691–0.984. The mean between-day variability was 36±65ms. The SRD was 130ms and 100% (9 out of 9 iSCI subjects) reached the SRD-criterion. If controls and iSCI subjects were grouped, the ICC was 0.979 (CI: 0.950–0.991) and the SRD was 96ms and 86% (19 out of 22 subjects) reached the SRD-criterion.

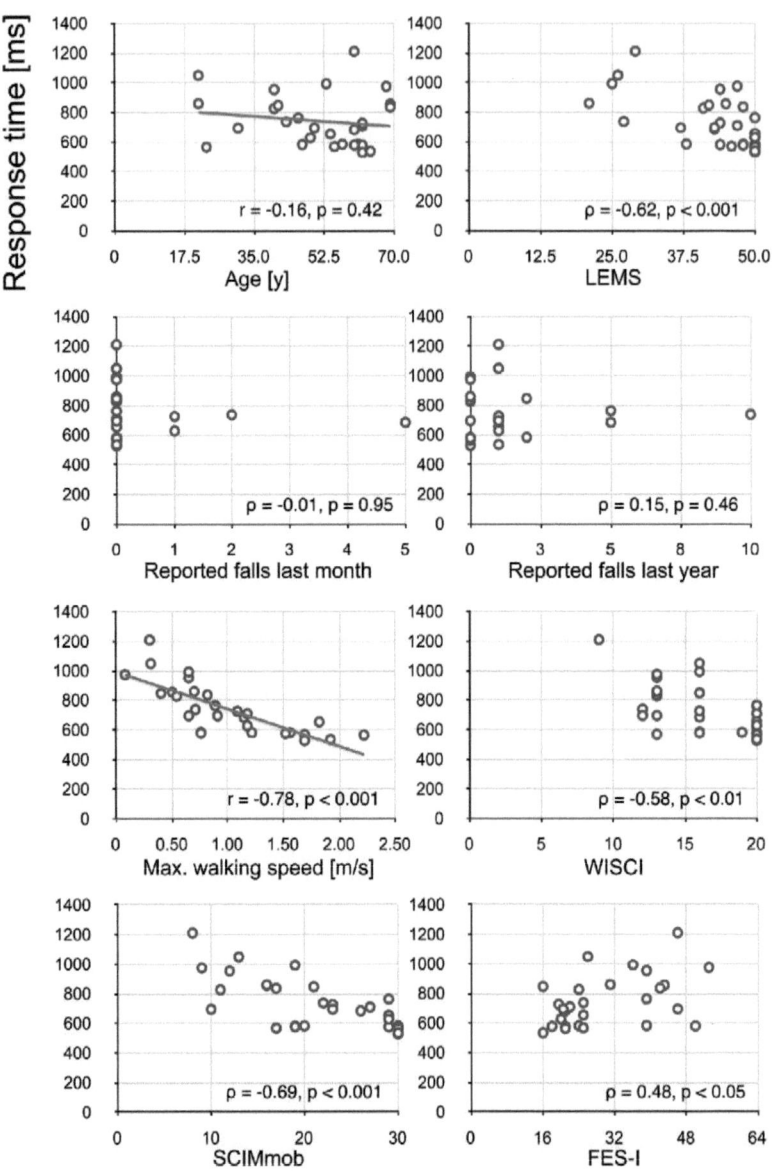

Figure 4.4: Correlations between choice response time and different characteristics in incomplete spinal cord injured subjects. Trendlines

are shown for parametric data only. LEMS = lower extremity motor score, max. = maximal, WISCI = Walking Index for Spinal Cord Injury, SCIMmob = mobility part of the Spinal Cord Independence Measure, FES-I = international version of the Falls Efficacy Scale.

4.5 Discussion

Fast response times are critical for maintaining balance when stepping and walking (van den Bogert et al., 2001; Maki and McIlroy, 1997). This might especially be relevant for the ambulating iSCI population because they already are prone to locomotor constraints. In general, CRT tests can shed some light on processes which involve decision making or action planning, which are not expected to be altered after iSCI, as well as motor command and quick, precise movement execution, which might be compromised after iSCI. The RET tries to address these cognitive and motor requirements needed when responding to continuously changing spatial and temporal information from the environment, during driving or stepping for example. Since there is no tool to assess CRT after iSCI up to now, the aim of this study was to validate this device for its possible use in this population.

The main findings were the following: Compared to controls, iSCI subjects have significantly slower CRTs, due to both prolonged reaction and movement times. Age does not seem to influence CRT as it does in healthy subjects. In iSCI subjects there were moderate to good correlations between CRT and several measures of function, but no significant association between CRT and reaction time and movement time, respectively. Retest reliability was high for both controls and iSCI subjects.

The large differences in CRT between iSCI subjects and controls can be explained by several factors:

(i) The prolonged movement time (+137ms) is likely due to the strength deficits of the iSCI subjects, as a strong relationship with the LEMS was observed. Indeed, our weakest 5 iSCI subjects with a LEMS of 20 to 30 had an average movement time of 535±127ms, whereas the 5 strongest subjects (maximal LEMS) reached an average of 227±35ms, and were practically as quick as the controls.

(ii) Several factors may account for the prolonged reaction time (+89ms). At first sight, it appears relatively straightforward, as conduction times of the corticospinal tract are often increased in iSCI subjects. For example, the for body-height normalized motor evoked potential latency of the tibialis anterior muscle could distinguish between controls and iSCI subjects with a sensitivity of 82% (van Hedel et al., 2007b), and Diehl et al reported a mean difference of 8ms in their sample (Diehl et al., 2006). Although these latencies reflect only the fastest corticospinal tract fibers, it still accounts only for about 10% of the observed difference in reaction time between iSCI subjects and controls. Additionally, in order to perform the stepping movement, subjects needed to shift the bodyweight from both legs to one leg, which might be prolonged especially in those subjects with diminished proprioception or lower extremity muscle strength. Furthermore, in some subjects with iSCI, hip flexor weakness might prolong the heel lift-off phase. As the heel lift-off distinguished between reaction and movement time, the initial movement time was recorded as the terminal reaction time. This appears especially the case in those iSCI subjects who have severely weakened muscles and slow maximal walking speeds, as can be seen from the asymptotic distribution of CRT against maximal walking speed (Figure 4.4).

Unlike in controls, age was not a dominant contributing factor to CRT in our sample of iSCI subjects. Apparently, the severity of the SCI was much more dominant, as significant relationships between CRT and muscle strength, as well as various functional capacity and performance measures, were observed. However, we failed to find correlations between functional measures and the sub domains of CRT. There were also no significant correlations between CRT and its own sub-domains, which suggests that the factors contributing to the variability of these sub-domains are not as straightforward and warrant further investigation in a larger sample.

Despite a moderate correlation between CRT and FES-I, there was no considerable association between CRT and the reported number of falls. This might be explained by the large number of sub-acute iSCI subjects in our sample (61%), whose injury occurred less then 8 months prior to the RET application and were considered non-fallers before their SCI. Therefore more studies are needed to study the relationship between prolonged CRT and fall risk in chronic iSCI subjects.

This device also could prove useful in patients with other neurologic conditions, like Huntington (Solomon et al., 2008), Multiple sclerosis (Marcotte et al., 2008) or Parkinson's disease (Mazzucchi et al., 1993) who show prolonged CRTs of the upper extremities. However, with the exception of stroke patients who have prolonged lower extremity CRTs (Melzer et al., 2009), information about lower extremity CRTs is missing. The RET could also shed some light on CRT in these patients, as they also show an increased risk for falling (Bilney et al., 2005; Peterson et al., 2008; King et al., 2010; Hyndman et al., 2002).

4.5.1 Study Limitations

We acknowledge that a drawback of this study is the simplified partitioning of CRT in reaction and movement time based on the heel lift-of movement. To overcome this limitation, we are currently performing a follow-up study, in which additional electromyographic recordings are being made, to more accurately identify the true reaction time. Also, the asymptotic correlation between CRT and maximal walking speed (Figure 4.4) suggests that obviously, a certain amount of function is a prerequisite to validly perform this test.

Results of the SRD calculations of the reliability data have to be interpreted with caution due to the sample size and the high standard deviations. Further studies are needed to calculate clinically applicable SRDs.

4.6 Conclusion

The RET is a valid and reliable tool to assess CRT of the lower extremities in healthy as well as ambulating iSCI subjects. It correlates considerably with several strength and ambulatory functional outcome measures in iSCI subjects.

4.7 Acknowledgement

We thank Johann Wanek for his technical support and his hours spent building the RET device. We gratefully acknowledge the individuals who participated in this study.

5 Motor deficits in well-rehabilitated people with incomplete spinal cord injury – a never-ending story?

Published in modified form in the journal *Archives of Physical Medicine and Rehabilitation*: Labruyère R, Zimmerli M, van Hedel JA. Slowed Down: Response Time Deficits in Well-Recovered Subjects With Incomplete Spinal Cord Injury. Arch Phys Med Rehabil. 2013;94:2020-6.

5.1 Abstract

Incomplete spinal cord injury leads to an impairment of motor function. In mildly affected subjects this motor function can be restored to a normative level with respect to locomotion and activities of daily living for instance. However, a structural damage of the neuromuscular system usually remains and so far it is unknown how these well-rehabilitated subjects perform in more demanding motor tasks. We therefore studied the ability of 15 subjects with incomplete paraplegia and clinically normal locomotor capabilities to perform a response time task with the lower limbs. They had to react as quickly as possible to a flashing light with a stepping movement. To investigate the loci of impairment we furthermore applied an upper limb response time task and transcranial magnetic stimulation. Hence, we were able to divide the complete response time into 4 separate parts: cortical time, conduction time, motor time and movement time. These findings were compared to those of 15 healthy controls. Results showed that well-rehabilitated subjects with incomplete spinal cord injury still suffered from deficits in conduction and movement time, whereas their cortical and motor times were essentially normal. Additionally these patients also suffered from delayed movement times of the upper limb, even if their injury was located in the thoracic or lumbar region. We conclude that well-rehabilitated patients with incomplete spinal cord injury still experience difficulties with quick and precise movements, which might have implications for translational researchers who aim to repair damaged spinal structures. Furthermore the combination of transcranial magnetic stimulation, electromyography and a response time task proved useful for the investigation of deficits in the course of executing fast movements and it could be applied to other patient groups as well. This is relevant since movement velocity is still not an established outcome measure to assess neurological impairment, although it can be used to detect subclinical deficits reliably and could be applied in the early detection of motor deficits.

5.2 Introduction

Spinal cord injury (SCI) is a diagnosis with a broad range of possible implications. On a spectrum from death to no consequences for future life, anything can be found, depending on extent and level of the lesion. SCI causes destruction and demyelination of axonal pathways as well as segmental spinal circuitries and therefore affects conduction of sensory and motor signals across the lesion site. Facilitation of recovery after SCI is a multidimensional approach. In this population, recovery of functions is usually accomplished by two mechanisms: 'adaptation' (e.g. application of an orthosis) and 'compensation' (e.g. training of new muscle synergies) (Curt et al., 2004). Rehabilitation is therefore mainly directed at strengthening and optimizing the preserved sensorimotor functions, training new movement strategies and using adaptive devices. However, only very few patients clinically recover completely from an SCI. A recent publication (van Middendorp et al., 2011) showed that one month post-injury, only 6 out of 1125 SCI patients (0.5%) were scored with an American Spinal Injury Association (ASIA) Impairment Scale (AIS, Marino et al., 2003) grade E, which stands for restitutio ad integrum with respect to motor score and sensory function (pin prick and light touch). This number is somewhat higher one year post-injury; Spiess et al. found 5 out of 284 SCI patients (1.8%) who were classified as AIS grade E (Spiess et al., 2009) and Marino et al. (Marino et al., 1999) showed that out of 1461 SCI patients 31 (2.1%) converted to Frankel grade E (precursor of the AIS, Frankel et al., 1969). Two earlier studies looking at long-term survival in SCI reported that 0% from 3179 patients (Frankel et al., 1998) and 2% from 4934 patients (De Vivo et al., 1991) were scored a Frankel grade E at discharge. The same articles however present much higher numbers of patients one year post-injury with AIS and Frankel grades D, i.e. patients with remaining minor motor or sensory deficits (ranging from 29.9% to 40.5%, Spiess et al., 2009; Marino et al., 1999). This indicates that a lot of well-rehabilitated patients with SCI might be suffering from remaining deficits, although they are well capable of performing regular activities of daily living (which has recently been shown for well recovered stroke patients, Planton et al., 2011).

In general, these patients are not considered to participate in clinical trials, because their spontaneous recovery, as quantified with recommended clinical tools such as the International Standards or the Spinal Cord Independence Measure (SCIM) (Steeves et al., 2007; Labruyère et al., 2010), is so strong that it easily could result in ceiling effects. We were therefore interested in documenting motor deficits in patients who had recovered extremely well from both a neurological and functional point of view. Some previous studies searched for sensitive motor measures that related to the neurological damage and remained affected in patients with iSCI, even after substantial clinical and functional recovery. A recent publication showed for example that maximal movement velocity was impaired and related well to corticospinal tract integrity, while impairments in strength as quantified with the ASIA motor score or static dynamometry did not correlate well (Wirth et al., 2008a). Another publication showed that also reaction times remained affected in patients with AIS grade D (Labruyère and van Hedel, 2011). Apparently reaction times and movement velocity might be sensitive indicators of even slight deficits in motor control, whereas for example accurate muscle coordination is not affected unlike in stroke patients (van Hedel et al., 2010).

In this study, we focus solely on the motor damage, as it is known that recovery of motor function is more important to patients with SCI than that of sensory function (Anderson, 2004). Having mentioned that, it must be noted that pain can severely impact quality and activities of daily living in chronic patients (Siddall, 2009).

Nevertheless, this influence appears less within the first year after SCI (van Hedel et al., 2011).

The aim of the present study was to analyze the physiological location of remaining motor deficits in well-rehabilitated subjects with SCI compared to a matched control group using a lower limb response time test combined with electromyographic measurements (EMG) and single-pulse transcranial magnetic stimulation (TMS). We use response times since they present an accurate method to measure central nervous system processing speeds (Huxham et al., 2001). Indeed, motor evoked potentials for example remain prolonged even in well-rehabilitated subjects with SCI, indicating that neurological recovery is only partial (Curt et al., 2008). We assume that by combining the results from these tests, we might predict how some translational approaches that target different sites of the damaged nervous system (from brain to effector muscle) might affect these results. This could indicate the potential use of this test battery to be used in Phase II clinical trials.

5.3 Methods

5.3.1 Participants

Subjects with an incomplete SCI (iSCI) were outpatients of our SCI centre, categorized as AIS grade D and with minimally reduced lower extremity strength (ASIA lower extremity motor score (LEMS) ≥ 48/50) and maximal scores in Spinal Cord Independence Measure (SCIM III, Itzkovich et al., 2007) and revised Walking Index for Spinal Cord Injury (WISCI II, Ditunno and Ditunno, 2001). Mean time since injury was 6.3 ± 5.5 years and 6 of the patients were prescribed antispastic medication. For more characteristics see Table 5.1. To ensure integrity of the upper limb, we only included patients with paraplegia (from T2 downwards).

Measure	Healthy (n = 15)	SCI (n = 15)	P-value
Subjects' characteristics			
Age, y	50.1 ± 12.3	50.2 ± 12.4	0.98
Female	5	5	n.a.
Systemic antispastic medication	n.a.	6	n.a.
Body height, m	170.7 ± 8.2	173.2 ± 10.4	0.30
Body weight, kg	69.7 ± 12.5	74.0 ± 18.0	0.28
Visual decimal acuity	1.1 ± 0.4	1.0 ± 0.3	0.47
Handedness	15 right-handed	15 right-handed	n.a.
Footedness	14 right-footed	15 right-footed	n.a.
Clinical characteristics and measures			
Lesion level	n.a.	T2 - T6: 1	n.a.
		T7 - T12: 7	n.a.
		L1 - L4: 7	n.a.
AIS grade	n.a.	all D	
LEMS	50	48.9 ± 0.8	< *0.001*
Knee extension strength, kg	37.7 ± 13.0	33.7 ± 14.6	0.14
Ankle dorsal flexion strength, kg	38.4 ± 16.0	31.3 ± 12.8	0.09
Ankle plantar flexion, kg	36.6 ± 6.1	31.8 ± 8.1	*0.02*
SCIM II	n.a.	100 ± 0	n.a
WISCI II	n.a.	20 ± 0	n.a
TUG, s	8.1 ± 0.9	9.2 ± 1.7	*0.001*

Table 5.1: Patient characteristics. Abbreviations: SCI = spinal cord injury; AIS = ASIA Impairment Scale; LEMS = Lower Extremity Motor Score; SCIM = Spinal Cord Independence Measure; WISCI = Walking Index for Spinal Cord Injury; TUG = Timed Up and Go test.

For all subjects, general characteristics and foot dominance (Chapman et al., 1987) were obtained by questionnaire. To assess strength, we applied the LEMS and measured isometric strength of three key muscle groups (knee extensors, ankle dorsiflexors and ankle plantarflexors) by using a force gauge (Mecmesin Limited, Slinfold, UK). As a measure of general function, we assessed the Timed Up and Go Test (TUG, van Hedel et al., 2005b). To exclude visual deficits, which might interfere with RET performance, we determined visual acuity (Bach, 1995). Normative values were obtained from healthy age- and gender-matched volunteers (Table 5.1).

5.3.2 Standard protocol approvals, registrations, and patient consents

The study protocol was approved by the local IRB of the Canton of Zurich. It followed the requirements of studies in humans as outlined in the Declaration of Helsinki and subjects gave written informed consent.

5.3.3 Devices

(1) To assess response times of the upper and lower limbs, we used the Reaction and Execution Test (RET, for a more detailed description see Labruyère and van Hedel, 2011). In short, it consists of a platform (57cm × 57cm × 3.5cm) containing 6 touch-sensors with a diameter of 1cm. Five target buttons are positioned in a semicircle 15cm from the tip of the starting position of the hand / foot. In the starting position, 1 button is located under the palm of the hand / heel of the foot. Next to each target button there is a corresponding blue light emitting diode (LED). Device control

software was written in LabVIEW 8.2.1 (National Instruments Corporation, Austin, Texas, USA).

(2) Corticospinal tract conductivity was assessed using TMS over the motor cortex. We used an angled figure-eight coil connected to a MagStim 200^2 (Magstim Company, Whitland, Wales). The optimal stimulation point was determined and the threshold was defined as the stimulator intensity where at least 5/10 pulses resulted in a response of 50μV above baseline (van Hedel et al., 2007b). Applied were single pulses at 1.2 times motor threshold. Motor evoked potential (MEP) responses were recorded from electrodes placed on the anterior tibial muscle (TA). This muscle was chosen, because it receives direct corticomotoneural projections (Brouwer and Ashby, 1992) and is directly involved in the RET. The onset latency was determined in an averaged signal over 5 MEPs. TMS and the RET were not applied at the same time since TMS influences response time (Day et al., 1989, Pascual-Leone et al., 1992).

5.3.4 Experimental setup

The RET was performed in a standing position between parallel bars with one foot at a time (the test was done for both feet). The other foot was comfortably placed in the lower corner of the platform. When an LED flashed up, the foot had to be positioned as quickly as possible on the associated target button. After this target button was pressed, the LED turned off and the subject moved the foot back to the starting position at a self-selected speed. EMG responses were simultaneously recorded from electrodes placed on the TA (2cm inter-electrode distance). As soon as the heel was placed back on the heel button, a new trial started.

All subjects performed at least 5 practice trials for each hand and each foot to familiarize with the task. During the experiment, the LEDs flashed up in a pseudo-randomized order in 6 randomized blocks. Each block consisted of 5 stimuli (per foot / hand: 30 stimuli) to ensure an even distribution over all target buttons.

To test the response time above the lesion, we applied the RET also for both hands (without EMG). Here we measured reaction time (time from appearance of the stimulus to release of the start button with the hand) and movement time (release of the start button with the hand to activation of the target button with the hand). For this test, subjects were equipped with a customized stiff glove (comparable to the shoe sole in the RET with the foot), to ensure comparable speed-accuracy trade-offs between upper and lower limb (Wickelgren, 1977).

5.3.5 Data analysis
For the upper limbs the 3 quickest reaction and movement time trials for each of the five target buttons were averaged for the left and right arm. The same was done for the lower limbs for the 3 quickest premotor, motor and movement time trials for each of the five target buttons. For each limb, these five values for each measure were then averaged into one reaction and one movement time for each

upper limb and one premotor, one motor and one movement time for each lower limb. These values were used for further analysis.

Reaction times (equal to premotor time plus motor time) quicker than 100 ms were considered false starts and not included in the response time analysis, just like each failed attempt, in which the target button was missed in the first attempt.

By combining the RET task with the neurophysiological EMG and TMS measurements, we were able to divide the total response time (from appearance of the RET stimulus to pressing the target button) into 4 time-windows (see Figure 5.1): (1) Cortical time: time between the appearance of the stimulus and the activation of the motor cortex. It was calculated by subtracting the MEP latency from the premotor time (i.e. time between the appearance of the stimulus and the first TA EMG activation, Botwinick and Thompson, 1966; Ballanger and Boulinguez, 2009). (2) Conduction time: time between activation of the motor cortex and TA EMG activation (i.e. MEP latency). (3) Motor time: time between the onset of TA EMG activity to release of the heel button with the foot (Botwinick and Thompson, 1966; Ballanger and Boulinguez, 2009). It was calculated by subtracting the premotor time from the reaction time (time from appearance of the stimulus to release of the heel button with the foot). (4) Movement time: time between the release of the heel button and pressing the target button with the foot.

5.3.6 Statistics

All variables were tested for normal distribution with the Shapiro-Wilk Test. Intra-group comparisons were done with the Paired Samples T Test (normally distributed data) and the Wilcoxon Signed Rank Test (not normally distributed data). Inter-group comparisons were done with the Independent Samples T Test (ISTT, normally distributed data) and the Mann-Whitney U Test (MWUT, not normally distributed data). Correlations were quantified with Pearson's rank correlation coefficients (r) for normally distributed data and with Spearman's Rho (ρ) for ordinal data. All the statistics were done using PASW Statistics 17 (IBM Company, New York, USA).

5.4 Results

Table 5.1 shows general characteristics and results of the additional measures of the 15 healthy controls and the 15 patients with SCI (4 patients had a LEMS of 50). Results for cortical time, conduction time, motor time and movement time for both groups assessed with the RET and TMS can be found in Figure 5.1. There was no significant difference for premotor time between controls and patients with SCI (209 ± 23 ms vs. 231 ± 48 ms, $p = 0.080$, MWUT). Distribution of reaction and movement times for the upper and lower limbs for both groups are depicted in Figure 5.2. Like movement times (Figure 5.1), reaction times of the lower limb were prolonged in SCI subjects (healthy: 283 ± 33 ms vs. SCI: 317 ± 52 ms, $p = 0.007$, MWUT). In contrast, reaction times of the upper limb were not different (healthy: 293 ± 38 ms vs. SCI: 298 ± 39 ms, $p = 0.690$,

MWUT), while the movement times were prolonged in the SCI subjects (healthy: 231 ± 37 ms vs. SCI: 292 ± 77 ms, p = 0.001, MWUT).

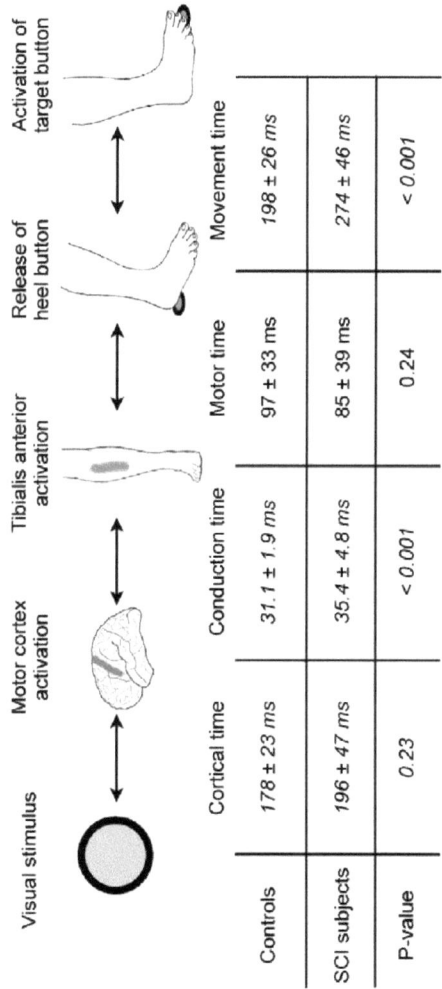

Figure 5.1: Comparison of cortical time, conduction time, motor time and movement time between the controls and the spinal cord injured (SCI) subjects.

There were no differences in mistakes between groups, neither for the upper limb (1.6 ± 1.3 vs. 1.8 ± 2.7, p = 0.460, MWUT) nor for the lower limb (1.7 ± 1.1 vs. 1.6 ± 1.6, p = 0.494, MWUT). There was no difference in any outcome measure between the patients that took antispastic medication and those who did not (p = 0.1 for TUG, MWUT, all other variables: p > 0.4, MWUT and ISTT).

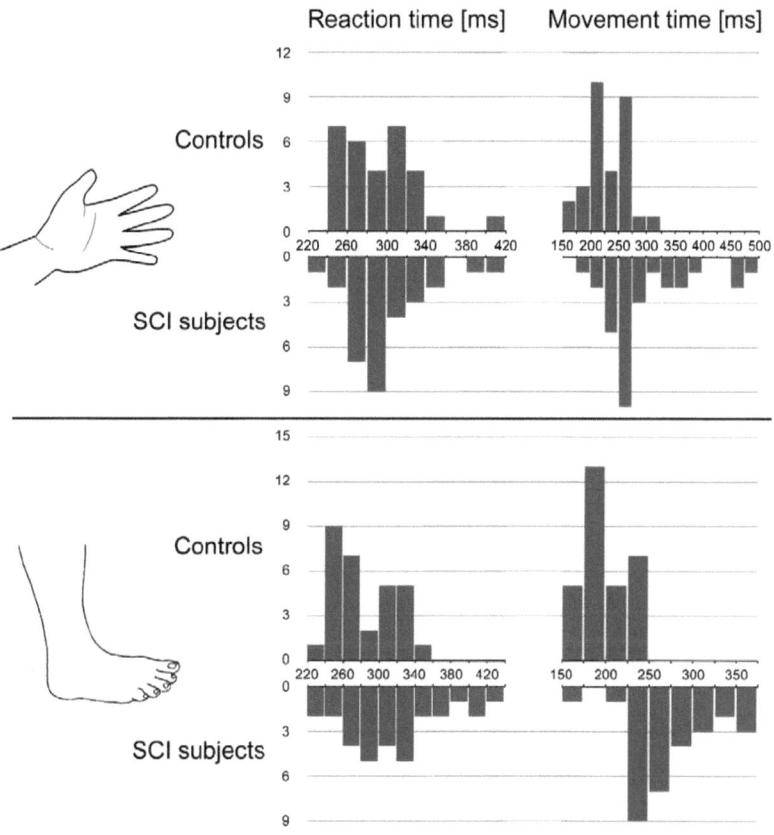

Figure 5.2: Distribution of reaction and movement times of controls and spinal cord injured (SCI) subjects displayed as histograms.

5.5 Discussion

An SCI usually has a considerable impact on the physical and psychological integrity of the person concerned. However, depending on extent and level of the lesion, the possibility of remission and reintegration into society as a functional walker exists. The results of this study show that well-rehabilitated chronic patients with an iSCI still have prolonged lower limb response times compared to healthy controls, which were mainly caused by prolonged conduction and movement times. Fast response times are essential for maintaining balance while stepping and walking (van den Bogert et al., 2002). Delayed response times could therefore among other factors be responsible for the increased risk of falling of ambulating patients with iSCI (Brotherton et al., 2007; Wirz et al., 2009).

In the following section we addressed the results for each of the 4 sites separately (as depicted in Figure 5.1) and suggest a potential application of the findings with respect to evaluating new experimental interventions.

5.5.1 Cortical time

In our study there was no significant difference in cortical time between healthy and patients with iSCI. At first sight, this appears relatively straightforward, as the brain seems not directly affected when the spinal cord gets injured. However, there have been a wide number of studies showing that cortical atrophy and / or reorganization occurs after complete as well as incomplete SCI (Green et al., 1999; Kokotilo et al., 2009; Wrigley et al., 2009; Freund et al., 2011). Several animal studies have demonstrated that cortical areas responsible for movement and sensation of intact body parts have a tendency to enlarge and invade areas responsible for a lost target after SCI (Raineteau and Schwab, 2001; Kokotilo et al., 2009). Accordingly, increases in volume of activation in the primary motor cortex in patients with SCI are associated with functional recovery (Jurkiewicz et al., 2007). Therefore, several groups have tried to improve functional motor recovery by intervening with the brain. However, studies dealing with repetitive TMS and transcutaneous direct current stimulation have led to inconsistent results (Belci et al., 2004; Jeffery et al., 2007; Kuppuswamy et al., 2011). As there were no differences in cortical time between the two groups, our results suggest that stimulation of the cortex is unlikely to result in increased motor function in patients with an incomplete paraplegia.

5.5.2 Conduction time

Patients with iSCI showed significantly slower conduction times measured with TMS. This has been demonstrated in earlier studies and it is also known that this latency-shift remains stable even in the case of symptom remission (Curt et al., 1998; van Hedel et al., 2007b). The reasons for the delayed motor evoked potentials lie in the disintegration of axons and disrupted pathways caused by SCI. Central long-distance regeneration does not occur spontaneously in the adult mammalian CNS because of a complex combination of factors both extrinsic and intrinsic to the lesioned neurons (Raineteau and Schwab, 2001). However, the majority of affected neurons survives (Beaud et al., 2008) and remains receptive to synaptic input (Tseng and Prince, 1996). Furthermore, existing regenerative sprouting of axons is a potential mechanism for functional reintegration of injured neurons into sensory–motor circuits (Bareyre et al., 2004). A combination of different experimental manipulations to induce regeneration is underway (for review, see Kwon et al., 2011a,b; Cadotte and Fehlings, 2011). However, it remains questionable whether regeneration in patients with incomplete lesions might induce faster conduction times, as the MEP latency reflects the integrity of the fastest well-myelinated fibers and it is unlikely that after an incomplete lesion, these improve. However, another therapeutic approach focuses on the remyelination of demyelinated fibers (Eftekharpour et al., 2007). Such an intervention, if successful, should actually result in improved MEP latencies and therefore we suggest that TMS might be used as a proof of principle for these therapies in patients with incomplete SCI.

5.5.3 Motor time

There was no significant difference for motor time between controls and patients with iSCI. It therefore seems that the muscles below the lesion can still be quickly activated. This might be explained by the fact that an iSCI leads to a shift toward the fast fiber population in the distal limb musculature below the lesion (Andersen et al., 1996; Crameri et al., 2002). This might compensate for the decline in the number of motor units that are usually caused by the damage of spinal motor neurons (Yang et al., 1990). However, as a consequence, the fatigability of the muscle might increase (Edgerton et al., 2002).

5.5.4 Movement time

Patients with SCI showed significant increases in movement time for the upper as well as lower limbs. Decreased maximal movement velocity of the lower limbs after incomplete SCI has been described recently (Wirth et al., 2008a) and it was shown that the recovery of MEP amplitudes went along with the improvement of maximal movement velocity. Furthermore, it has been confirmed that an iSCI affects movement velocity more compared to isometric strength (Wirth et al., 2008a). Indeed, after an iSCI, the cross-sectional area of muscles below the level of lesion becomes reduced, although the remaining presence of neural inputs to the muscle results in more modest atrophy compared to patients with complete SCI (Shah et al., 2006). Nevertheless, the voluntary drive might not recruit all motor neurons that supply lower limb muscles, thereby reducing maximal strength (Shields, 2002), as seen in our sample (Table 5.1).

Improvements in strength, however, occur after iSCI and can be induced by specific strength training (Gregory et al., 2007; Curt et al., 2008; Jayaraman et al., 2008) or functional electrical stimulation (Granat et al., 1993). Initially, it is likely that besides some spontaneous neurological recovery (for example spontaneous peripheral sprouting from innervated to denervated muscle fibers (Marino et al., 1994) training-induced changes affect first the neural drive behind these muscles followed by muscle hypertrophy after sustained training. Assessing movement velocity therefore remains a more accurate measure to document impairments in muscle activations compared to manual muscle testing or even isometric dynamometry.

The reasons for increased movement time of the upper limbs in our patients with paraplegia remain unclear, as their hands were not affected by the SCI. This was in line with a publication showing reduced upper limb response times in paraplegic patients performing time-critical tasks in a driving-simulator (Lings, 1991). Perhaps trunk instability might play a role, as despite that these patients were very well recovered, complex tasks requiring much balance like the TUG were slightly but significantly prolonged in the SCI subjects. Furthermore, as the RET was performed in a standing position counter-forces had to be generated by the trunk and leg musculature, which might have affected upper extremity movement time. However, further studies are needed to shed light on the underlying mechanisms of decreased maximal movement velocity of the upper limbs. There is also no literature on how to optimize maximal movement velocity in well recovered patients with SCI.

5.5.5 Generalizability to other patient groups

Response time and maximal movement velocity are reported to be affected in various other patient groups. Especially patients with neurological conditions such as Huntington (Solomon et al., 2008), multiple sclerosis (Marcotte et al., 2008), stroke (Melzer et al., 2009; Chang et al., 2006), Parkinson's disease (Mazzucchi et al., 1993) or cerebellar disease (Küper et al., 2011) are prone to impaired movement times. Even otherwise healthy former athletes who suffered a concussion show reduced maximal movement speeds (De Beaumont et al., 2009). With the combination of TMS, EMG and a response time task, deficits in the course of executing fast movements can be detected and approximately localized. This is relevant since movement velocity is still not an established outcome measure to assess neurological impairment, although it can be used to detect subclinical deficits reliably and could be applied in the early detection of motor deficits. Furthermore, the ability to perform rapid movements is a marker for longevity (Metter et al., 2005).

5.5.6 Study limitations

We acknowledge that our approach to calculate cortical time has some methodological flaws. TMS elicits a descending volley by directly or transsynaptically activating corticospinal cells at or close to the soma (Petersen et al., 2003), whereas during the RET probably an interneural spike train density-dependent mechanism applies. However, Leocani et al. showed that corticospinal activation in a response time task happens in series and not in parallel with stimulus processing and decision-making (Leocani et al, 2000). Therefore the fragmentation in processing and conduction time seems to be appropriate. Furthermore, we didn't differentiate between central and peripheral neural conduction velocity, thus more studies are needed to investigate differences in well-rehabilitated patients with SCI. At last, we did not assess spasticity in patients with SCI as a possible factor that could influence movement velocity.

5.6 Conclusion

Even well-rehabilitated patients with SCI who are fully reintegrated into society experience difficulties in performing quick and precise movements. This can have an impact on their ability to quickly adapt to environmental challenges. Origin of these difficulties is mainly found in the muscles, but also corticospinal approaches could be effective to overcome these deficits.

6 Lower extremity strength training outperforms robot-assisted gait training in walking-related outcome measures in moderately ambulating subjects with incomplete spinal cord injury

Published in modified form in the journal *Journal of NeuroEngineering and Rehabilitation*: Labruyère R, van Hedel JA. Strength training versus robot-assisted gait training after incomplete spinal cord injury: a randomized pilot study in patients depending on walking assistance. J Neuroeng Rehabil. 2014;9;11(1):4.

6.1 Abstract

Objective: To compare changes in several walking-related outcome measures due to robot-assisted gait training (RAGT) and lower extremity strength training in subjects with chronic incomplete spinal cord injury.

Subjects: Nine chronic ASIA Impairment scale grade D (sensory-motor incomplete) subjects were randomly assigned to the intervention groups. They had moderate walking ability and time since spinal cord injury was ≥ 1 year.

Intervention: Group 1 received 16 sessions of RAGT (45min each) within 4 weeks followed by 16 sessions of lower extremity strength training (45min each) within 4 weeks. Group 2 received the same interventions in reversed order.

Outcome measures: Assessment of several walking-related measures such as walking speed under different circumstances, balance, strength, gait efficiency and symmetry and several questionnaires that assess activities of daily living and risk of falling. Data was collected at baseline, between the interventions after 4 weeks, at the end of the interventions and at the follow-up six months after the end of the second intervention.

Results: Lower extremity strength training led to significantly greater improvements compared to RAGT. Especially in all walking tests the superiority of strength training was striking. Only in the Walking Index for Spinal Cord Injury and the maximal medio-lateral amplitude of postural sway the RAGT intervention led to greater improvements than strength training.

Limitations: The participants might have been physically too strong for RAGT and strength training was much more customizable compared to RAGT. Furthermore, sample size was very low.

Conclusion: To improve walking-related outcome in moderately ambulating incomplete spinal cord injured subjects, strength training seems to be more effective compared to RAGT.

6.2 Introduction

In the 1980s it has been shown that spinalized cats recover significant locomotor capability after treadmill training with partial bodyweight support (Barbeau and Rossignol, 1987). Based on these results the concept of manually assisted body weight-supported treadmill training (BWSTT) was extended to spinal cord injured humans (Visintin and Barbeau, 1989). Thereafter, BWSTT developed to an acknowledged evidence-based clinical approach (Barbeau, 2003) and it is applied in subjects with all kinds of neurological movement disorders, especially stroke and incomplete spinal cord injury (iSCI) (Dietz et al., 1995; Hesse et al., 1994). However, the technical progress enabled letting robots do part of the work and there were several robotic gait devices being developed. They allow a prolonged training duration, a high number of steps per training session (repetition) and facilitate the work of the therapists. These driven gait orthoses, like for example the Lokomat (Hocoma AG, Volketswil, Switzerland) (Colombo et al., 2001; Riener et al., 2010) have been successfully introduced in more and more rehabilitation and research clinics to treat and analyze individuals with a locomotor dysfunction (Hesse et al., 2003). Together with locomotor-unspecific strength training (ST), BWSTT, be it robotic or manual, builds the basis of neurorehabilitation in many settings worldwide.

On the basis of clinical experience and the results of BWSTT studies it may seem logical that task-specific locomotor training, such as robot-assisted gait training (RAGT) has more advantages compared to an unspecific muscle ST intervention. The main reason is that task-specific training provides locomotion-relevant afferent input (especially loading of the limbs and hip extension, Dietz and Harkema, 2004) to the spinal central circuitries that are responsible for generating rhythmic stepping behavior (Bouyer, 2005). But also unspecific ST of the lower limbs might lead to functional improvements after stroke or iSCI, since there is a correlation between ambulatory capacity and strength of certain leg muscles (Richards and Olney, 1996; Kim et al., 2004).

Still, there is literature that shows a superiority of task-specific locomotor training over ST in subjects with stroke (Hesse et al., 1995; Laufer et al., 2001; Sullivan et al., 2007). However, in this case the results of stroke patients cannot necessarily be extrapolated to patients with iSCI. Recent studies showed that after an iSCI, complex muscle coordination and motor programs appear intact, while muscle strength is affected (Wirth et al., 2008c; van Hedel et al., 2010). This is unlike stroke, where complex muscle coordination was disturbed even in the "unaffected" leg (van Hedel et al., 2010). However, these studies investigated single joint movement tasks and it therefore remains questionable whether these findings can be translated into more functional movements, such as walking. That is why our aim was to compare gait-related outcomes of task-unspecific lower extremity ST and task-specific locomotor training in patients with a chronic iSCI, especially since recent publications indicated that different task-specific approaches all seem to perform equally well (Mehrholz et al., 2008; Field-Fote et al., 2005; Nooijen et al., 2009).

There already have been some training studies with robots in patients with iSCI. Wirz et al. for example found improvements in gait velocity and endurance after RAGT in chronic iSCI subjects (Wirz et al., 2005). However, a control group was lacking and it remains uncertain whether walking-specific RAGT results in a better walking ability than rather unspecific leg muscle ST. To shed light on this issue we applied several walking tests, most of which cover walking speed in different forms, like the 10m Walk Test (10MWT, van Hedel et al., 2009). Furthermore, we assessed symmetry of gait, which has been shown to improve after locomotor-specific training in subjects with iSCI (Field-Fote et al., 2005). It is an important marker for the quality of gait and an accurate indicator of changes in the walking pattern, even on a sub-clinical level (Benedetti et al., 1999). There is evidence that gait symmetry also improves after lower extremity ST in stroke subjects (Teixeira-Salmela et al., 2001). To cover the risk of falling after iSCI, which is largely increased (up to 75%) (Brotherton et al., 2007; Wirz et al., 2009) we measured balance, since they are related (Maki et al., 1994) and balance is considered very important for functional ambulation after iSCI (Scivoletto, 2008). Furthermore, Barbeau and Visintin showed that manual BWSTT improves balance in stroke subjects (Barbeau and Visintin, 2003). However, as patients are strongly fixated in the robot, it remains questionable whether balance becomes trained during RAGT, as recently discussed for patients with stroke (Mayr et al., 2007; Hidler et al., 2009).

Overall, the aim of this study was to compare the effects of RAGT and ST on outcome measures of walking and balance in chronic iSCI subjects.

6.3 Methods

6.3.1 Participants

Four women and 5 men (mean age = 59.5 ± 11.0 years) participated in this study. All had experienced an iSCI at least 12 months earlier (mean time since injury = 4.1 ± 4.7 years). None of them had an orthopedic, neurological or psychiatric disease, except for the SCI.

Characteristics can be found in Table 6.1. Participant enrollment started in March 2009 and the final participant completed training in April 2011. To be considered for inclusion, subjects had to be between the age of 18 and 70 with a chronic incomplete spinal cord injury (time after injury > 1 year). Patients had to be rated as grade C or D on the American Spinal Cord Injury Association (ASIA) Impairment Scale (AIS) (Marino et al., 2003). These patients are sensorimotor incomplete. While in AIS grade C patients more than half of specific key muscles below the lesion are graded a manual muscle score below 3, at least half of the muscles below the lesion in AIS grade D patients is scored 3 or stronger (Marino et al., 2003). The motor level of lesion should be between C4 and T11 to exclude patients with peripheral lesions. Furthermore, participants had to be unable to walk without at least moderate assistance at the time of inclusion (i.e. a score of less than 6 in the "mobility outdoors" item of the latest version of the Spinal Cord Independence Measure [SCIM], Itzkovich et al., 2007). Cognitive capacity to follow simple verbal instructions was necessary and tested with the Mini Mental State Examination (minimal score to be reached was 26, Folstein et al., 1975).

Exclusion criteria were similar to those provided by the manufacturer of the Lokomat System (Hocoma AG, Volketswil, Switzerland): body weight greater than 130 kg, body height greater than 2 m, leg length difference greater than 2 cm, osteoporosis, instable fracture in lower extremity, restricted range of motion or presence of decubitus ulcer of lower extremity. Also, any of the following diseases limiting training led to exclusion of the study: arthritis causing pain while

ID	IG	Age (years)	Height (cm)	Weight (kg)	Sex	Months p. injury	Level of lesion	Etiology	AIS	WISCI
P01	2	69	178	68	m	16	C4	trauma	D	13
P02	1	69	178	80	m	13	T8	tumor	D	16
P03	1	43	163	54	w	84	T11	trauma	D	12
P04	2	60	166	75	w	21	T4	abscess	D	16
P05	1	60	179	92	m	44	T11	hern	D	9
P06	2	41	161	48	w	189	C6	trauma	D	16
P07	1	53	183	85	m	29	C5	hern	D	13
P08	2	67	164	89	w	27	C5	hern	D	16
P09	1	69	179	93	m	26	C4	trauma	D	16

Table 6.1: Characteristics of the participants. Abbreviations: ID = identification; IG = Intervention group; AIS = ASIA Impairment Scale grade; WISCI = Walking Index for Spinal Cord Injury; m = man; w = woman; hern = herniation; C = cervical; T = thoracic.

stepping; dyspnea or angina on moderate exertion; limited walking endurance due to cardiopulmonary or other diseases. Prevalence of other neurological or orthopedic injuries and medical diseases which may limit exercise participation or impair locomotion (e.g. serious infection; severe orthostatic hypotension or uncontrolled hypertension, congestive heart failure, pain while weight-bearing) as well as severe metabolic diseases, epilepsy, pre-morbid ongoing major depression or psychosis were additional exclusion criteria. Patients were asked to maintain their regular medication scheme and inform the principal investigator about any changes or extraordinary events.

The research database of our hospital was screened for possible candidates. A total of 97 entries were found to approximately match the inclusion and exclusion criteria and these subjects were contacted and invited. Out of 10 subjects who were screened on site, 1 did not meet the inclusion criteria. The other 9 people were willing to participate and they all finished the intervention including the follow-up measurements. The Consolidated Standards of Reporting Trials (CONSORT) diagram can be seen in Figure 6.1.

6.3.2 Ethics

All subjects gave written informed consent and the study protocol was approved by the ethics committee of the Canton of Zurich, Switzerland. Additionally, the trial was registered at www.clinicaltrial.gov (NCT01087918).

6.3.3 Training protocol and rehabilitation device

This study was a single-blind randomized cross-over clinical trial comparing RAGT and conventional ST in chronic iSCI subjects. Subjects were assigned to either group 1 or group 2. Group 1 received 16 sessions of RAGT within 4 weeks followed by 16 sessions of ST within 4 weeks. Group 2 received the same intervention in reversed order. Before, in between and after the interventions and 6 months after the last training session, assessments took place (Figure 6.2).

The "state-of-the-art" ST focused on the most important leg muscles needed for walking. The RAGT could be considered more than "state-of-the-art" as besides the clinically applied position controlled mode, two additional interactive modes allowed the patient to interact with the robot and to interact with the robot and the treadmill

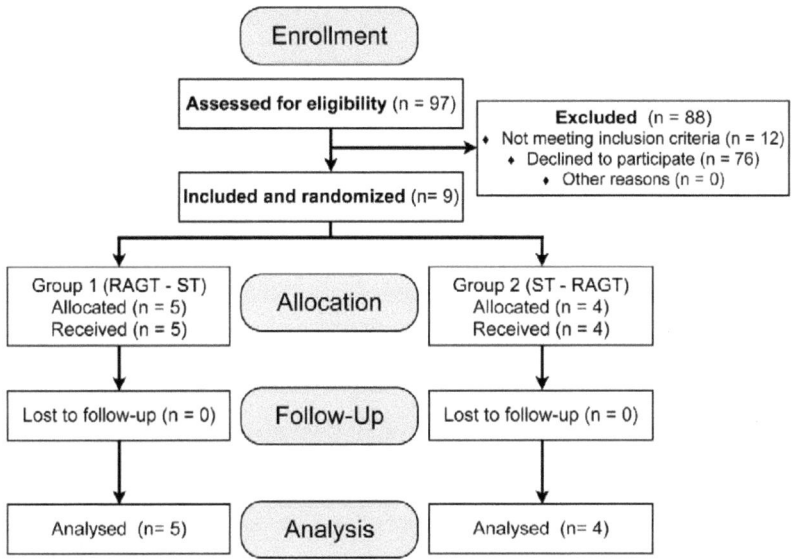

Figure 6.1: Consolidated Standards of Reporting Trials diagram. Abbreviations: RAGT = robotic assisted gait training; ST = strength training.

speed (the interactive modes were based on path control rather than position control, see Vallery et al., 2009a,b for more information). This enabled matching the training to the patients' capabilities like it was done in ST. Additionally, by applying the adequate training mode, the patients were forced to actively participate, whereas in earlier clinical trials they theoretically could just be passive (Nooijen et al., 2009; Field-Fote and Roach, 2011). The RAGT was performed with the Lokomat System. More detailed information about the Lokomat system can be found in the related publications (Colombo et al., 2001; Riener et al., 2010). Briefly summarized, the Lokomat comprises two actuated leg orthoses that are attached to the patient's legs. Passive foot lifters can be added to induce ankle dorsiflexion during swing phase. Patients are connected via a harness to a bodyweight support system. This allows relieving a definable amount of the patient's weight on the legs and therefore makes performing leg movements easier.

Training duration per session was 45min (actual training time) for both interventions. The first session of RAGT focused on adjusting the system to the patient. To allow patients to familiarize with the system, training started with approximately 30% body-weight support and a treadmill speed between 1 and 2 km/h. All patients initially started training using foot lifters to ensure foot clearance during swing phase thereby preventing stumbling. If control and strength of ankle dorsiflexion improved, the tension of the foot lifters was decreased until volitional dorsiflexion was sufficient to remove the foot lifters. In subsequent sessions, training intensity was increased progressively by changing walking speed, level of body-weight support, robotic support or by applying the next higher training mode. The amount of body-weight support was adjusted individually in order for the patients to achieve adequate knee extension during stance phase and toe clearance during swing phase. ST consisted of the same amount of training as the RAGT. Just like the RAGT it was executed under the supervision of a movement scientist. The training was particularly aimed at lower limb muscle strength. Subjects with tetraplegia also received ST of the upper extremity if it promised to improve ambulation according to recent findings (Wirz et al., 2006).

6.3.4 Outcome measures

Selected items (demographic and SCI-specific data of interest, Table 6.1) of the International Spinal Cord Injury Core Data Set (De Vivo et al., 2006) were collected and the motor score of the neurological examination according to the ASIA International Standards (Marino et al., 2003) was evaluated (upper extremity motor score in subjects with tetraplegia only). Furthermore, we applied the SCIM to assess independence and several outcome measures of walking and balance. All outcome measures were applied according to Figure 6.2.

Walking

Preferred and maximal walking speeds during the 10MWT (van Hedel et al., 2009) were evaluated. The subjects were instructed to walk at their preferred and maximal speed. The 10MWT was performed with a "flying start" (i.e., while the subject walked about 14m, the time was measured for walking the intermediate 10m). Details about the standardization have been previously described (van Hedel et al., 2008). To test the subjects' ability to adapt their gait to several circumstances, we developed the Figure of Eight Test (FET) with different conditions (Figure 3.1). The figure of eight had a length of 10m. It consisted of 2 adjacent circles with a radius of each 160cm. Path width was 80cm to ensure that the test could also be done with a walker. The path that had to be followed was marked with tape and delimited with cones (Figure 3.1). All subjects started and ended their walking at least 1.5m outside the figure of eight to minimize acceleration and deceleration effects. The outcome measure was time needed for one lap for every condition. The stopwatch was started as soon as the first foot crossed the midline and it was stopped as the first foot crossed the dashed midline again after one lap. All trials were recorded on video to control times offline. The FET consisted of 6 different conditions mimicking several specific demands of functional walking:

- FET preferred: This provided insight in difficulties with turning – which might increase demands for balance – in contrast to the straight-walking 10MWT.
- FET maximal: FET at maximal safe walking speed.
- FET vision: Subjects wore glasses simulating cataract (blurred view, 10% of normal vision). This emphasized dependence on vision.
- FET obstacle: Two obstacles (one in each curve, Figure 3.1) with a width of 60cm, height of 10cm and a depth of 7cm had to be overstepped. The height of the obstacle corresponded to an average curb in Switzerland.
- FET foam: Subjects wore foamed soles under their shoes. This emphasized dependence on the proprioceptive system.
- FET dual task: During walking, a number of questions had to be answered as quickly as possible. This provided information about the amount of "automaticity" of walking, i.e. the attentional demand required for walking.

Except for FET maximal, subjects were directed to walk at self-selected speed corresponding to their preferred comfortable walking speed in everyday life. All walking tests were performed on a flat, smooth, nonslippery surface, with no disturbing factors and the tester walked next to the subject for reasons of safety and measurement accuracy. Results of all walking tests were converted to walking speed (m/s).

Furthermore, we applied the Revised Walking Index for Spinal Cord Injury (WISCI, Ditunno and Ditunno, 2001) to assess, which kind of assistive devices the subjects were using to cover 10m and we estimated energy expenditure with the Physiological Cost Index (PCI, Ijzerman et al., 1999). The PCI was assessed on a treadmill. First, subjects stood for 2 minutes and mean heart rate of the last 10s was used as resting heart rate. Then they walked for 3 minutes with the same speed they walked in their first preferred 10MWT. Then it was calculated as follows: PCI = (steady-state heart rate − resting heart rate)/ambulatory velocity. Finally, we measured gait symmetry by comparing lengths of stance and swing phases of every single leg (by dividing stance time [in % of whole step] right by stance time left) with portable insoles. If the value was ≥ 1, it was inverted to ensure comparability. Gait symmetry was measured in 8 subjects only due to infrastructural issues.

Balance
We used the Berg Balance Scale (BBS, Berg et al., 1992) as a performance-based measure of balance. It consists of 14 subtests and has a maximal score of 56 points. As a marker of static balance, we measured the maximal medio-lateral amplitude of the center of pressure movement over 30s on a force plate (subjects were asked

to stand as still as possible, fixate a given object with their eyes and the distance between their feet was 10cm) (Rogers et al., 2003). The test was done twice and the best try counted. To assess fear of falling while performing different activities of daily living, we applied the international version of the Falls Efficacy Scale (FES-I, Yardley et al., 2005).

6.3.5 Data analysis

We analyzed two basic aspects in this study; on the one hand we compared the effects of RAGT with the effects of ST (irrespective of which group the participants were in) and on the other hand we were interested whether the order of interventions played a role (group 1 vs. group 2). For the first aspect the usual statistical method would be an analysis of variance, however due to the low number of participants, we cannot assume normal distribution of data. We therefore used effect size indices (Cohen's d, Cohen, 1988) and nonparametric testing. We calculated effect sizes of each separate intervention by subtracting pre- from post-interventional values (for outcome measures where a larger number represents a better performance; vice-versa for outcome measures where a lower number represents a better performance) and dividing them by the pre standard deviation (Dunlap et al., 1996). Additionally, we applied Wilcoxon tests to find differences from pre to post intervention. For the difference of RAGT vs. ST, we calculated the effect sizes by taking the difference between the mean improvements and dividing them by the pooled standard deviation (as we hypothesized that RAGT might lead to better results, we subtracted the difference after

ST from the difference after RAGT) (Rosnow et al., 1996).

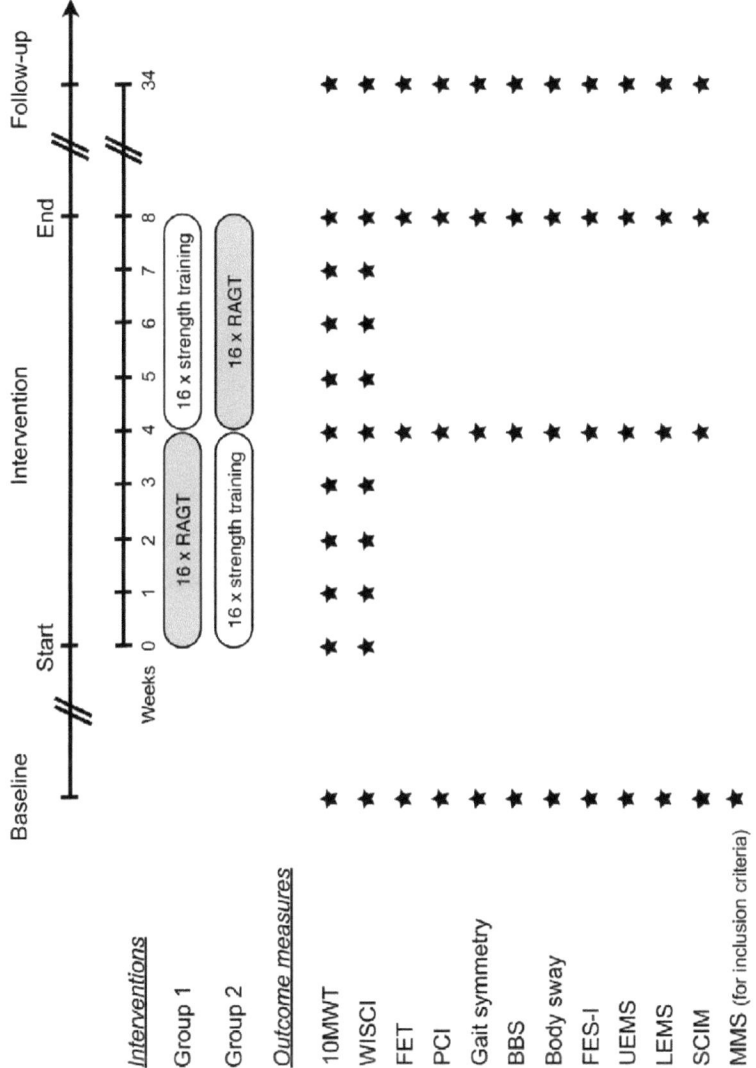

Figure 6.2: Application scheme of outcome measures. Abbreviations: RAGT = robotic assisted gait training; 10MWT = 10m

Walk Test; WISCI = Walking Index for Spinal Cord Injury; FET = Figure-Eight-Test; PCI = Physiological Cost Index; BBS = Berg Balance Scale; FES-I = Falls Efficacy Scale – International Version; UEMS = upper extremity motor score; LEMS = lower extremity motor score; SCIM = Spinal Cord Independence Measure; MMS = Mini Mental State Examination.

Furthermore, we applied Mann-Whitney U Tests to find differences between both interventions. According to Cohen (Cohen, 1988), effect sizes of d = 0.2 are considered small, d = 0.5 are medium and d ≥ 0.8 are large. For the nonparametric tests, we applied a significance level of $p \leq 0.05$. For detecting differences between group 1 and group 2, we calculated effect sizes as described above (Dunlap et al., 1996) and applied Mann-Whitney U Tests.

6.4 Results

All participants completed both interventions and no adverse events occurred. Overall, ST led to better results compared to RAGT, especially in the walking tests, where the maximal 10MWT and the FET with foamed soles yielded significant results (Table 6.2).

6.4.1 Walking

ST led to higher improvements in all walking tests compared to RAGT (Table 6.2 and Figure 6.3). Walking speed in the maximal 10MWT, maximal FET and FET with foamed soles improved significantly after ST whereas no significant improvements after

RAGT were found (Table 6.2). Only two subjects improved their walking ability determined by the WISCI. One subject (P04) who used two crutches before the training series could walk without any assistive devices after RAGT (WISCI score improved from 16 to 20). Another subject who used a walker at inclusion improved to using two crutches after RAGT (from 13 to 16) and improved further after ST, where he used one cane only (from 16 to 19). The PCI improved after ST (from 0.84 ± 0.74 beats/m to 0.65 ± 0.41 beats/m) while it deteriorated after RAGT (from 0.76 ± 0.40 beats/m to 0.88 ± 0.70 beats/m). Gait symmetry approached 1 (optimal symmetry) after both interventions (from 0.91 ± 0.18 to 0.93 ± 0.13 after RAGT and from 0.93 ± 0.13 to 0.96 ± 0.10 after ST).

6.4.2 Balance

With respect to balance measures, the BBS improved significantly after ST (from 42.7 ± 14.0 to 45.4 ± 14.7 points), but not after RAGT (from 43.3 ± 14.7 to 44.4 ± 14.7 points). The maximal medio-lateral amplitude of postural sway decreased after RAGT (from 1.76 ± 1.13cm to 1.41 ± 0.80cm), whereas it remained almost constant after ST (from 1.86 ± 0.91cm to 1.82 ± 1.01cm). The FES-I showed almost no changes (from 26.6 ± 8.7 to 26.4 ± 9.2 after RAGT and from 25.6 ± 7.3 to 25.1 ± 5.5 after ST).

Outcome measure (n=9, unless otherwise indicated)	RAGT	Interventions, separately P-value (Wilcoxon)	ST	P-value (Wilcoxon)	Interventions, comparison RAGT vs. ST	P-value MWUT
10MWT preferred	0.19	0.26	0.33	0.08	-0.22	0.51
10MWT maximal	0.03	0.72	0.64	**0.01**	*-0.82*	**0.03**
FET preferred	0.02	0.67	0.24	0.26	-0.52	0.44
FET maximal	0.06	0.44	0.24	**0.01**	*-0.93*	0.11
FET vision	0.03	0.73	0.10	0.40	-0.25	0.67
FET obstacles	-0.02	1.00	0.24	0.09	*-0.84*	0.09
FET foam	0.00	0.81	0.30	**0.02**	*-1.11*	**0.04**
FET dual task	0.14	0.34	0.21	0.17	-0.08	0.80
WISCI	0.31	0.18	0.13	0.32	0.33	0.67
Gait symmetry (n=8)	0.12	0.61	0.27	0.21	-0.36	0.87
PCI	-0.30	0.16	0.26	0.16	-0.65	0.08
Sway (force plate)	0.31	0.09	0.05	0.61	0.47	0.14
BBS	0.08	0.11	0.20	**0.02**	*-0.87*	0.11
FES-I	0.02	0.68	0.08	0.62	-0.10	1.00
UEMS (n = 5)	0.16	0.71	0.48	0.46	-0.29	0.75
LEMS	0.09	0.11	0.15	**0.03**	-0.31	0.61
SCIM	0.10	0.34	0.16	0.07	-0.27	0.93

Table 6.2: Effect sizes for all outcome measures of separate interventions and for the comparison of both interventions. For the comparison of both interventions, positive effect sizes indicate superiority of RAGT and negative effect sizes superiority of ST. D = 0.2 is a weak effect, d = 0.5 is a medium effect and d ≥ 0.8 is a strong effect. All effect sizes ≥ 0.8 are italic, all p-values ≤ 0.5 are bold. Abbreviations: RAGT = robotic assisted gait training; ST = strength training; MWUT = Mann-Whitney U Test; 10MWT = 10m Walk Test; pref = preferred; max = maximal; FET = Figure-Eight-Test; WISCI = Walking Index for Spinal Cord Injury; PCI = Physiological Cost Index; BBS = Berg Balance Scale; FES-I = Falls Efficacy Scale – International Version; UEMS = upper extremity motor score; LEMS = lower extremity motor score; SCIM = Spinal Cord Independence Measure.

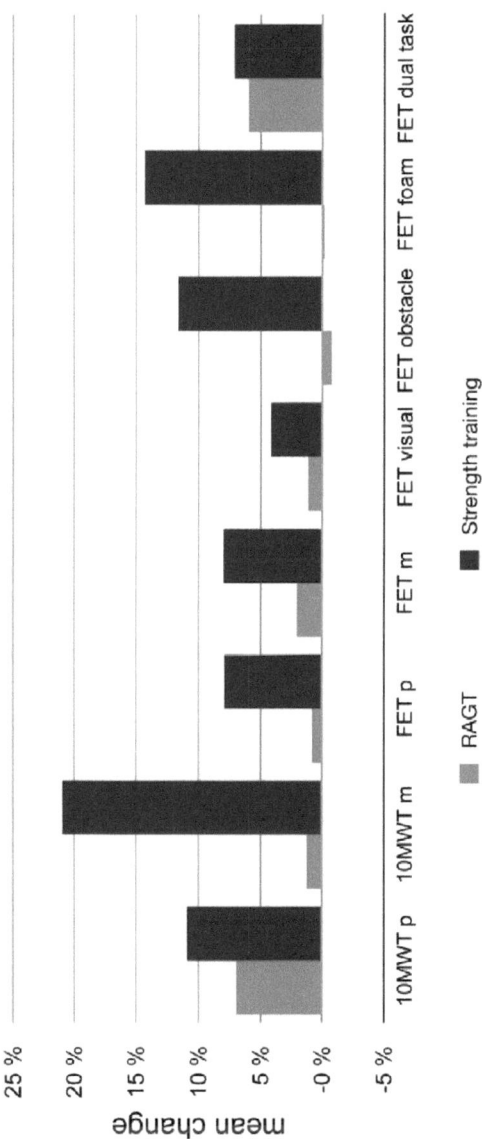

Figure 6.3: Mean improvements in walking speed after RAGT and strength training for different conditions. Abbreviations: RAGT =

robotic assisted gait training; 10MWT = 10m Walk Test; p = preferred; m = maximal; FET = Figure-Eight-Test.

6.4.3 Additional measures

Motor scores improved more after ST (from 42.4 ± 2.1 to 43.4 ± 2.6 for the upper extremities and from 40.4 ± 6.6 to 41.4 ± 6.9 for the lower extremities) compared to RAGT (from 43.0 ± 2.6 to 43.4 ± 3.2 for the upper extremities and from 40.9 ± 7.5 to 41.6 ± 7.3 for the lower extremities). The SCIM improved more after ST (from 87.9 ± 8.1 to 89.2 ± 7.9) compared to RAGT (from 88.4 ± 7.9 to 89.2 ± 7.6).

6.4.4 Group differences

Age and time since injury were comparable in both groups. The maximal 10MWT and the maximal medio-lateral amplitude of postural sway improved significantly different between group 1 and group 2 (Table 6.3).

6.5 Discussion

We had hypothesized that due to the activation of locomotor spinal central circuitries, RAGT would lead to greater improvements in different walking-related outcome measures compared to ST. This was not supported by the results. ST was associated with greater improvements in most of the outcome measures, but there were only few significant results.

Outcome measure	Effect size for group comparison	P-value
Age	n.a.	1.00
Time since injury	n.a.	0.81
10MWT preferred	-0.32	0.46
10MWT maximal	*-1.99*	**0.05**
FET preferred	0.33	0.81
FET maximal	0.56	0.62
FET vision	0.56	0.54
FET obstacle	-0.71	0.46
FET foam	-0.40	0.46
FET dual task	0.55	0.81
WISCI	0.08	1.00
Gait symmetry[a]	*1.24*	0.10
PCI	1.01	0.14
Sway (force plate)	*-1.61*	**0.03**
BBS	-0.07	1.00
FES-I	*0.80*	0.54
UEMS[b]	-0.22	0.78
LEMS	*-1.19*	0.13
SCIM	-0.70	0.43

Table 6.3: Effect sizes and p-values of the Mann-Whitney U Test for intervention order. Group 1 (n = 5) received robotic-assisted gait training followed by strength training, group 2 (n = 4) received the interventions in reversed order. Positive effect sizes indicate higher improvements in group 1 and negative effect sizes higher improvements in group 2. D = 0.2 is a weak effect, d = 0.5 is a medium effect and d ≥ 0.8 is a strong effect. All effect sizes ≥ 0.8 are italic, all p-values ≤ 0.5 are bold. [a] n = 5 for group 1 and n = 3 for group 2. [b] n = 2 for group 1 and n = 3 for group 2. Abbreviations: 10MWT = 10m Walk Test; FET = Figure-Eight-Test; WISCI = Walking Index for Spinal Cord Injury; PCI = Physiological Cost Index; BBS = Berg Balance Scale; FES-I = Falls Efficacy Scale –

International Version; UEMS = upper extremity motor score; LEMS = lower extremity motor score; SCIM = Spinal Cord Independence Measure.

6.5.1 Walking

The results of the 10MWT at preferred and at maximal speed, already point out that RAGT is not superior compared to lower extremity ST. Especially the maximal 10MWT led to significant improvements after ST, whereas it practically remained constant after RAGT. This was unexpected, since the walking speed in the Lokomat at the end of the intervention exceeded over-ground walking speed in the maximal 10MWT in 6 of 9 subjects. We therefore specifically trained fast walking. However, Field-Fote et al. already reported that treadmill speed in RAGT does not seem to be an essential factor for locomotor outcomes in subjects with iSCI (Field-Fote et al., 2005). Kim et al. showed on the other hand that muscle strength correlates with walking speed (Kim et al., 2004). Since LEMS improved significantly after ST, this might have led to higher walking speeds. It seems that maximal walking speed is not an appropriate outcome measure to detect changes in locomotion after RAGT. Also preferred walking speed did not change significantly after RAGT and this is in line with results of studies published earlier (Field-Fote et al., 2005; Field-Fote and Roach, 2011). However, the main difference to these studies lies in the fact that in our study, patients were forced to actively participate in the Lokomat, thus eliminating passiveness as a reason for the inferiority of RAGT. Yet there are also studies where RAGT led to improvements of preferred walking speed (Wirz et al., 2005; Hornby et al., 2008). The efficacy of RAGT seems to depend on the initial walking function of the participant. Those with lower initial walking speeds are likely to profit more from this intervention compared to those with higher walking speeds (Wirz et al., 2005; Field-Fote et al., 2005). In the study of Wirz et al. the preferred walking speed of all participants before intervention was around 0.4m/s (Figure 3 in Wirz et al., 2005) and 0.45m/s in the study of Hornby et al. (Table 3 in Hornby et al., 2008) whereas our subjects walked considerably faster when they entered the study (0.57 ± 0.20m/s, all but two walked ≥ 0.44m/s). Nevertheless, none of the patients reached the 0.9m/s that were suggested as threshold for community ambulation for subjects with paraplegia (Cerny et al., 1980). The results of the outcome measures of walking were reflected in the results of the SCIM where improvements were also greater after ST. Changes were only achieved in the mobility (indoors and outdoors) subscale of the SCIM and can therefore be seen as improvements of functional walking ability.

Walking speed in all conditions of the FET showed more improvements after ST compared to RAGT. This consistency is remarkable and shows that the results of the 10MWT are not just of statistical value, but indicate that ST really seems to have a greater impact on walking function than RAGT. The finding of van Hedel et al. in subjects with iSCI that strength is predominantly affected, while accurate muscle activation remains largely unaffected (van Hedel et al., 2010), might explain, why an unspecific strength training actually performed better compared to a specific locomotor training in our participants. This is also reflected in the more or less constant improvement in walking speed these subjects experienced after ST, irrespective of which FET condition we applied (except for the FET maximal).

The WISCI improved several levels in two subjects. This is noteworthy, since a recent paper described that already an improvement of 1 level in the WISCI is clinically relevant (Burns et al., 2011). However, these improvements do not seem attributable to one of the two interventions. It was rather due to improved self-confidence that these two subjects gained over the 2 months of training (personal observation of the authors, no data).

The PCI deteriorated after RAGT and improved after ST, but there was a big inter-individual variability that hindered drawing conclusions. Differences between resting and walking heart rate were in general very small indicating that walking for three minutes at preferred speed was not a very energy-demanding load in our sample. Additionally, low walking speeds compared to those of the non-disabled population led to big statistical data spread. Therefore the PCI must be looked at critically in this population as already noted by Ijzerman et al. (Ijzerman et al., 1999).

With the assessment of gait symmetry, we wanted to detect possible changes in gait biomechanics, since an earlier study had demonstrated improvements in gait symmetry due to RAGT (Field-Fote et al., 2005). However, gait symmetry did not significantly change and this is in line with results of another study (Nooijen et al., 2009). It must be noted though that all but one (P05) subjects had no relevant strength differences between their right and left leg.

6.5.2 Balance

Our balance measures showed equivocal results. ST led to significant improvements in the BBS. This could be expected, since this had already been shown in other populations, such as stroke patients (Weiss et al., 2000) or elderly (Hess et al., 2005). However, static balance on the force plate did practically not change and this has also been shown in a broad range of publications in non-disabled subjects (for review, see Orr et al., 2008). After RAGT, it was the other way round. While the BBS improved only slightly, the maximal medio-lateral amplitude of postural sway decreased almost significantly. While the influence of RAGT on the BBS has been investigated in an earlier publication in stroke subjects (led to significant increase, Hidler et al., 2009), its effect on static balance has herewith been investigated for the first time. At first sight, one would think that balance could not really be trained in the Lokomat, because subjects are firmly attached to the device and they are secured from falling by different mechanisms (body weight support, hand rails, foot lifters). Nevertheless, it seems as if training in the Lokomat has positive effects on static and performance-based balance. Further studies are needed to clarify this issue.

6.5.3 Group differences and limitations

We found large effect sizes for some outcome measures with respect to the group that participants were randomized to. Due to the low number of patients in each group, this analysis was even more susceptible to individual variability than the comparison of RAGT vs. ST. This can be well seen in the FET, where different conditions led to high effect sizes in favor of group 1 as well as in favor of group 2. We therefore assume, that randomization order did not play a role in the development of outcome measures in this study, despite significant results. However, it points out to the limitations of this study. Sample sizes are known to be rather small in exercise training studies involving subjects with chronic SCI (Martin Ginis et al., 2005). Our study unfortunately is no exception. Larger sample sizes would have allowed for more sophisticated statistical methods and greater statistical power. Additionally, the generalizability of our findings is limited to people with the narrowly defined inclusion and exclusion criteria applied in this study. As mentioned above, it might be that the subjects who participated in this study were clinically too good for the Lokomat. However, we tried to accommodate this flaw by applying different training modes and there were only two patients who were able to acceptably manage the most difficult training mode, where interaction with the treadmill speed was possible. Nevertheless, ST is customizable to a much higher extent compared to RAGT. The therapist is able to specifically address weaknesses that result in straight improvements of function.

Furthermore, optimal training dosage still is unknown. The number of training sessions and the duration of each training session were chosen according to clinical experience and no participant complained about physiological overload.

At last, during RAGT we did not focus on a specific aim. Usually, we tried to let the patients walk as fast as possible, but as in the clinical application, we also focused on lowest possible robotic and body weight support.

6.6 Conclusion

A locomotor-unspecific ST of the lower extremities leads to better results in walking-related outcome measures compared to a task-specific RAGT in subjects with chronic iSCI with limited ambulatory function. Especially outcome measures of walking speed showed a clear advantage of the much more customizable ST.

7 Effects of robot-assisted gait training and lower extremity strength training on motor evoked potentials and response times of the leg in moderately ambulating subjects with incomplete spinal cord injury

7.1 Abstract

Objective: To compare changes in motor evoked potentials and response times due to robot-assisted gait training (RAGT) and lower extremity strength training (ST) in subjects with chronic incomplete spinal cord injury.

Subjects: Nine chronic ASIA Impairment scale grade D (sensory-motor incomplete) subjects were randomly assigned to the intervention groups. They had moderate walking ability and time since spinal cord injury was ≥ 1 year.

Intervention: Group 1 received 16 sessions of RAGT (45min each) within 4 weeks followed by 16 sessions of lower extremity ST (45min each) within 4 weeks. Group 2 received the same interventions in reversed order.

Outcome measures: Motor evoked potentials of the anterior tibial muscle were elicited with transcranial magnetic stimulation. Furthermore, we assessed lower extremity response times, which were divided into reaction and movement times. Data was collected at baseline, between the interventions after 4 weeks, at the end of the interventions and at the follow-up six months after the end of the second intervention.

Results: Latencies of motor evoked potentials remained constant around 38ms, irrespective of which intervention was performed. Response times also stagnated in the course of RAGT (from 788 ± 194ms to 786 ± 171ms) as well as ST (from 770 ± 166ms to 753 ± 156ms).

Conclusion: Neither locomotor-unspecific ST nor locomotor-specific RAGT led to improvements in MEP latencies or response times of the lower extremities in our sample of subjects with chronic iSCI with limited ambulatory function. It remains unclear, whether the low sample size and the high variability masked possible changes in response time.

7.2 Introduction

International numbers on the incidence of spinal cord injury (SCI) vary between 10 to 83 persons per million every year (Wyndaele and Wyndaele, 2006). More than 50% of these patients suffer from a sensory-motor incomplete lesion, that is, sensory and/or motor function is partially preserved below the level of lesion (Wyndaele and Wyndaele, 2006; National Spinal Cord Injury Statistical Center Facts&Figures, 2011). One of the primary goals of rehabilitating patients with incomplete SCI (iSCI) is regaining ambulatory function (Ditunno et al., 2008). To achieve this aim, usually extensive training is necessary. Nowadays, this training clinically often consists of a combination of task-specific exercise, i.e. locomotor training, and task-unspecific exercise, like strength training (ST) to allow patients to become as independent as possible. For locomotor training, especially two approaches have prevailed: Manually assisted body weight-supported treadmill training (BWSTT) and robot-assisted locomotor training (RAGT). BWSTT was developed in animal studies and it could be shown that spinalized cats recovered significant locomotor capability after treadmill training with partial bodyweight support (Barbeau and Rossignol, 1987). Thereafter BWSTT was extended to human patients and found its way to therapy of subjects with iSCI (Visintin and Barbeau, 1989; Dobkin, 1999). However, especially training with severely affected patients is considerably exertive for therapists. This was the main reason why RAGT was originally developed. In BWSTT therapists have to facilitate the desired movements of paretic and occasionally spastic limbs and they also need to guarantee the safety of the patients and prevent them from falling. Therefore, usually 2-3 therapists are needed for the training of a single patient. With the development of driven gait orthoses, like for example the Lokomat (Hocoma AG, Volketswil, Switzerland) (Colombo et al., 2001; Riener et al., 2010), this number can be reduced to 1. Furthermore, RAGT allows for longer training times (high number of repetitions) and a precise biomechanical control of movement. Nevertheless, both approaches are applied and since their introduction a wide range of studies has been published (for review, see Mehrholz et al., 2008; Hicks and Martin Ginis, 2008).

Since research on neural plasticity highlighted the ability of the central nervous system to reorganize and relearn, both approaches were thought to make a more valuable contribution to gait rehabilitation compared to unspecific training. This is confirmed by findings that task specificity plays a key role in motor learning.

Indeed, a recent study in subjects with stroke demonstrated greater improvements in walking speed after a task-specific intervention (BWSTT) compared to a task-unspecific intervention (resisted leg cycling) (Sullivan et al., 2007) and this premise was suggested to be translatable to iSCI (Fouad and Tetzlaff, 2011). However, other recent studies showed that after an iSCI, complex muscle coordination and motor programs appear intact, while muscle strength is affected (Wirth et al., 2008c; van Hedel et al., 2010). This is unlike stroke, where complex muscle coordination was disturbed even in the "unaffected" leg (van Hedel et al., 2010). This suggests that the changes due to training after iSCI might happen rather on a spinal than a cortical level. On the other hand, Winchester and colleagues found changes in supraspinal activation patterns after RAGT (Winchester et al., 2005). However it is not known, whether these activation patterns are actually meaningful for the specific rehabilitation of subjects with iSCI or if they are regular patterns not different from those of healthy subjects. It therefore remains unclear in how far spinal characteristics change after specific and unspecific locomotor training. To gain further insights in the spinal mechanisms we therefore investigated, whether a task-specific RAGT has different effects compared to an unspecific ST on outcome measures reflecting descending pathways. We investigated corticospinal tract conductivity via the latencies of motor evoked potentials of the anterior tibial muscles. Furthermore response times of the lower extremities were assessed, since they present an accurate method to measure central nervous system processing speeds (Huxham et al., 2001).

7.3 Methods

Since data in this chapter originates from the same study as data in chapter 6, the description of *participants* (chapter 6.3.1), *ethics* (chapter 6.3.2), *training protocol and rehabilitation device* (chapter 6.3.3) and *data analysis* (chapter 6.3.5) is identical. Therefore, information can be found in the respective chapters.

7.3.1 Main outcome measures

(1) To assess latencies of the anterior tibial muscle, we applied transcranial magnetic stimulation (TMS) over the motor cortex according to a protocol described earlier (van Hedel et al., 2007b): In short, we used an angled figure-eight coil connected to a MagStim 200^2 (Magstim Company, Whitland, Wales). The optimal stimulation point was determined and the threshold was defined as the stimulator intensity where at least 5/10 pulses resulted in a response of 50µV above baseline. Single pulses were applied at 1.2 times motor threshold. Motor evoked potential (MEP) responses were recorded from electrodes placed on the anterior tibial muscle. This muscle was chosen, because it receives direct corticomotoneural projections (Brouwer and Ashby, 1992). The onset latency was determined in an averaged signal over 5 MEPs per leg. Additionally, we recorded motor threshold (in % of stimulator output) as a measure of corticospinal excitability.

(2) To assess response times of the lower limbs, we used the Reaction and Execution Test (RET, for a more detailed description, see Labruyère and van Hedel, 2011). In short, it consists of a

platform (57cm × 57cm × 3.5cm) containing 6 touch-sensors with a diameter of 1cm. Five target buttons are positioned in a semicircle 15cm from the tip of the starting position of the foot. In the starting position, 1 button is located under the heel of the foot. Next to each target button there is a corresponding blue light emitting diode (LED). The heel button serves to divide response time into reaction time, the time from flashing of the LED to release of the heel button, and movement time, the time from release of the heel button to activation of the target button. Device control software was written in LabVIEW 8.2.1 (National Instruments Corporation, Austin, Texas, USA).

The RET was performed in a standing position between parallel bars with one foot at a time (the test was done for both feet). The other foot was comfortably placed in the lower corner of the platform. When an LED flashed up, the foot had to be positioned as quickly as possible on the associated target button. After this target button was pressed, the LED turned off and the subject moved the foot back to the starting position at a self-selected speed. As soon as the heel was placed back on the heel button, a new trial started. All subjects performed at least 5 practice trials for each foot to familiarize with the task. During the experiment, the LEDs flashed up in a pseudo-randomized order in 6 randomized blocks. Each block consisted of 5 stimuli (per foot: 30 stimuli) to ensure an even distribution over all target buttons.

7.3.2 Additional measures

Selected items (demographic and SCI-specific data of interest, Table 6.1) of the International Spinal Cord Injury Core Data Set (De Vivo et al., 2006) were collected. To control the development of muscle strength, we measured the lower extremity motor score of the neurological examination according to the ASIA International Standards (Marino et al., 2003). Additionally, the maximal isometric voluntary force (L-Force) and mechanical stiffness (L-Stiff, as an estimate for spasticity) of extensors and flexors of the knee and of the hip within the Lokomat were measured (for further details, see Riener et al., 2010).

All outcome measures were applied before, in between and after the interventions and 6 months after the last training session.

7.4 Results

All participants completed both interventions and no adverse events occurred.

There were no significant effects of either intervention on main outcome measures (Table 7.1).

MEP latency of the anterior tibial muscles remained constant in the course of both interventions (mean latency: from 38.2 ± 7.0ms to 38.6 ± 7.0ms after RAGT and from 38.0 ± 6.5ms to 38.4 ± 7.5ms after ST). Also motor threshold remained rather constant (mean threshold: from $71.1 \pm 21.4\%$ to $69.2 \pm 22.4\%$ after RAGT and from $70.3 \pm 23.1\%$ to $71.2 \pm 21.7\%$ after ST). Response times did not change after RAGT (mean response time: from 788 ± 194ms to 786

± 171ms) whereas they slightly improved after ST (from 770 ± 166ms to 753 ± 156ms). Effect size for mean response time (RAGT vs. ST) was d = -0.25. If response time was split up into reaction and movement time of each leg, we got the following picture: Right and left reaction times remained constant after RAGT (right: from 396 ± 53ms to 393 ± 81ms and left: from 423 ± 97ms to 425 ± 90ms) and also after ST (right: from 381 ± 57ms to 374 ± 53ms and left: from 408 ± 100ms to 404 ± 67ms). The same was true for movement times for RAGT (right: from 372 ± 166ms to 359 ± 107ms and left: from 384 ± 130ms to 395 ± 115ms) as well as ST (right: from 361 ± 109ms to 344 ± 100ms and left: from 390 ± 111ms to 383 ± 131ms).

7.4.1 Additional measures

The lower extremity motor scores improved more after ST (from 40.4 ± 6.6 to 41.4 ± 6.9) compared to RAGT (from 40.9 ± 7.5 to 41.6 ± 7.3). As indicated by effect sizes, L-Force (flexors and extensors combined) improved slightly after RAGT for hip (from 46.2 ± 16.0kg to 50.6 ± 12.2kg) as well as knee (from 36.3 ± 12.1kg to 39.0 ± 12.7kg), while after ST it remained rather constant (hip: from 45.0 ± 10.6kg to 46.5 ± 11.2kg; knee: from 38.0 ± 9.8kg to 36.7 ± 11.4kg).

Outcome measure	Interventions, separately				Interventions, comparison	
	RAGT	P-value (Wilcoxon)	ST	P-value (Wilcoxon)	RAGT vs. ST	P-value MWUT
MEP latency right	0.02	0.58	0.01	0.75	0.05	0.67
MEP latency left	-0.15	0.17	-0.15	0.21	-0.04	0.93
Mot. threshold right	0.11	0.14	-0.05	0.66	*0.80*	0.32
Mot. threshold left	0.05	0.47	-0.03	0.59	0.45	0.25
Reaction time right	0.06	0.68	0.12	0.68	-0.06	0.80
Reaction time left	-0.02	0.86	0.04	0.59	-0.14	0.63
Movement time right	0.08	0.78	0.16	0.19	-0.07	0.73
Movement time left	-0.08	0.68	0.07	0.59	-0.45	0.49
LEMS	0.09	0.11	0.15	**0.03**	-0.31	0.61
L-Force hip	0.27	0.34	0.15	0.68	0.26	0.55
L-Force knee	0.22	0.44	-0.13	0.48	0.66	0.30
L-Stiff hip	0.15	0.81	-0.13	0.64	0.39	0.83
L-Stiff knee	0.13	0.37	0.00	0.77	0.24	0.73

Table 7.1: Effect sizes for all outcome measures of separate interventions and for the comparison of both interventions. For the comparison of both interventions, positive effect sizes indicate superiority of RAGT and negative effect sizes superiority of ST. According to Cohen, d = 0.2 is a weak effect, d = 0.5 is a medium effect and d ≥ 0.8 is a strong effect. All effect sizes ≥ 0.8 are italic, all p-values ≤ 0.5 are bold. Abbreviations: RAGT = robotic assisted gait training; ST = strength training; MWUT = Mann-Whitney U Test; MEP = motor evoked potential; Mot. = motor; SI = stimulation intensity of transcranial magnetic stimulation; LEMS = lower extremity motor score; L-Force = isometric voluntary force measured in the Lokomat; L-Stiff = mechanical stiffness measured in the Lokomat.

Furthermore, L-Stiff did not considerably change, neither after RAGT (hip: from 0.66 ± 0.42 to 0.60 ± 0.34; knee: from 0.20 ± 0.15 to 0.18 ± 0.15) nor ST (hip: from 0.56 ± 0.33 to 0.61 ± 0.37; knee: from 0.18 ± 0.16 to 0.18 ± 0.12).

Outcome measure	Effect size for group comparison	P-value
Age	n.a.	1.00
Time since injury	n.a.	0.81
Mean MEP latency	0.77	0.33
Mean motor threshold	-0.65	0.31
Mean reaction time	*1.03*	0.46
Mean movement time	0.52	0.62
LEMS	*-1.19*	0.13
L-Force hip	*-0.95*	0.14
L-Force knee	-0.22	1.00
L-Stiff hip	0.55	0.62
L-Stiff knee	0.50	0.46

Table 7.2: Effect sizes and p-values of the Mann-Whitney U Test for intervention order. Group 1 (n = 5) received robotic-assisted gait training followed by strength training, group 2 (n = 4) received the interventions in reversed order. Positive effect sizes indicate higher improvements in group 1 and negative effect sizes higher improvements in group 2. According to Cohen, d = 0.2 is a weak effect, d = 0.5 is a medium effect and d ≥ 0.8 is a strong effect. All effect sizes ≥ 0.8 are italic. Abbreviations: MEP = motor evoked potential; LEMS = lower extremity motor score; L-Force = isometric voluntary force measured in the Lokomat; L-Stiff = mechanical stiffness measured in the Lokomat.

7.4.2 Group differences

Age and time since injury were comparable in both groups and there were no significant differences in outcome measures between group 1 and group 2 (Table 7.2). However, due to the low number of participants, there were some considerable effect sizes when comparing groups.

7.5 Discussion

This study was performed to investigate the effects of locomotor-specific and locomotor-unspecific training on outcome measures concerning the spinal cord. Results show that in our sample, neither training intervention had a considerable effect. However, this has to be interpreted carefully against the background of low statistical power due to the sample size.

7.5.1 Spinal conductivity

Latency of MEPs did not change, neither after RAGT nor ST. This is in contrast to results of an earlier study, where improvement of MEP latencies after stroke could be demonstrated (Platz et al., 2005). However, latencies changed only on the affected side and it can therefore be assumed that improvement occurred cortically (Platz et al., 2005). An iSCI also affects cortical regions (Freund et al., 2011), but motor programs seem to be spared unlike after stroke (van Hedel et al., 2010). Since the MEP latency reflects the integrity of the fastest well-myelinated fibers, and remyelination of the spinal cord after an injury does not happen without external intervention

(Eftekharpour et al., 2007), it remains questionable whether training in patients with iSCI might induce faster conduction times at all.

7.5.2 Response time

Neither response time nor its sub-categories reaction and movement time changed substantially in the course of any given intervention. The small improvement of 17ms after ST cannot be considered relevant, since the smallest real difference in this population is 130ms (Labruyère et al., 2011). We had hypothesized that response times would decrease after RAGT, since it specifically addresses descending pathways, therefore theoretically offering the possibility to enhance voluntary control of the foot. Also an improvement after ST would have been plausible, since response time and strength correlate (Labruyère et al., 2011) and LEMS showed a significant improvement after ST. Furthermore, Delmonico et al. demonstrated that ST improves maximal movement velocity (Delmonico et al., 2005) and therefore decreases movement time. Since there were almost no significant improvements in outcome measures, maybe participants did not respond to the interventions as expected. Especially for the RAGT, subjects were possibly too good already at the beginning of the intervention. It therefore remains unclear, whether subjects profited too less from the interventions to show improvements in such specific measurements or if differences would be detected in a larger sample with lower variability.

7.5.3 Additional measures

Our measures of strength showed opposing results. The lower extremity motor score improved after ST, while L-Force, which is measured directly in the Lokomat device, increased more after RAGT. However, measurement of L-Force highly depends on the relative position of the subject in the Lokomat. A small displacement can already change torques at hip and knee joints of the device substantially, leading to moderate intra-rater reliability (Bolliger et al., 2008). The same holds true for the L-Stiff measurement, where no differences were found.

7.5.4 Group differences and limitations

We found large effect sizes for some outcome measures with respect to the group that participants were randomized to. However, statistically there were no significant differences. Due to the low number of patients in each group, effect size analysis is susceptible to individual responders.

This points out to the limitations of this study. Sample sizes are known to be rather small in exercise training studies involving subjects with chronic SCI (Martin Ginis et al., 2005). Our study unfortunately is no exception. Larger sample sizes would have allowed for more sophisticated statistical methods and greater statistical power. Furthermore, we included patients with diverse etiologies as well as a mixture of paraplegic and tetraplegic patients and the generalizability of our findings is limited to people with the narrowly defined inclusion and exclusion criteria applied in this study. As mentioned above, it might be that the subjects who participated in this study were clinically too good for the Lokomat. However, we tried to accommodate this flaw by applying different training modes and there were only two patients who were able to acceptably manage the most difficult training mode, where interaction with the treadmill speed was possible. Nevertheless, ST is customizable to a much higher extent compared to RAGT. The therapist is able to specifically address weaknesses that result in straight improvements of function.

Furthermore, optimal training dosage still is unknown. The number of training sessions and the duration of each training session were chosen according to clinical experience and no participant complained about physiological overload.

At last, during RAGT we did not focus on a specific aim. Usually, we tried to let the patients walk as fast as possible, but as in the clinical application, we also focused on lowest possible robotic and body weight support.

7.6 Conclusion

Neither locomotor-unspecific ST nor locomotor-specific RAGT led to improvements in MEP latencies or response times of the lower extremities in our small sample of subjects with chronic iSCI with limited ambulatory function.

8 Pain alleviation after robot-assisted gait training in patients with incomplete spinal cord injury

Published in modified form in the journal *Journal of NeuroEngineering and Rehabilitation*: Labruyère R, van Hedel JA. Strength training versus robot-assisted gait training after incomplete spinal cord injury: a randomized pilot study in patients depending on walking assistance. J Neuroeng Rehabil. 2014;9;11(1):4.

8.1 Abstract

Robotic assisted gait training (RAGT) has widely spread over the last few years in neurorehabilitation facilities. It complements conventional physical therapy and alleviates manual assisted body weight-supported treadmill training (BWSTT). Nowadays, it is frequently being used to improve functional ambulation after incomplete spinal cord injury (iSCI). There is literature showing that single sessions of BWSTT have positive effects on pain perception and physiological well being in this population. However, it is unknown, whether this is also true for RAGT. To obtain more insight into this problem, a small prospective clinical trial was performed. Eight patients (mean age: 58.3 ± 11.0 years) with chronic iSCI and different pain types performed 16 sessions of RAGT with the device 'Lokomat'. They participated in a structured pain interview before and after the intervention and rated their current pain before and after each training session on a 100 mm visual analog scale (VAS). Results showed that in these patients, pain intensity was only moderate, but still RAGT significantly reduced it over time (regression coefficient r = -0.33, p = 0.04). Additionally, we found a trend towards short-term pain relieving effects from before to after each training session. Therefore, we suggest that regular RAGT can lead to a reduction of moderate pain intensity after chronic iSCI.

8.2 Introduction

Besides muscle paralysis, individuals with spinal cord injury (SCI) are highly susceptible to many secondary health issues. Chronic pain is such an issue and it can affect physical functioning beyond levels attributable to the SCI alone (Martin Ginis et al., 2003; Rintala et al., 1998). Approximately, two thirds of the SCI population experience chronic SCI-related pain (Richards et al., 1980; Siddall et al., 2003). Several mechanisms are thought to be responsible for chronic pain (Eide, 1998) and it may express above, at and below the level of lesion (Siddall, 2009). The results of a survey of 200 individuals with SCI illustrate the possible impact of chronic pain: 25% of the respondents described their pain as severe to extreme, 44% stated that their pain interfered with daily activities, and 37% of the individuals with higher level injuries and 23% of the individuals with lower level injuries reported that they would trade pain relief for loss of bladder, bowel or sexual function (Nepomuceno et al., 1979). Since pharmacological treatments to restore normal sensory processing have not prevailed for all patients (Heutink et al., 2011), the search for alternative possibilities that might relief pain is ongoing.

One such possibility is physical activity, which has been shown to be rather effective in treating pain (Hicks et al., 2005). It is an essential part of rehabilitative strategies after traumatic injuries of the nervous system (Behrman and Harkema, 2007; Edgerton et al., 2004) and several studies suggest that physical activity might improve sensory function (Hutchinson et al., 2004). A commonly applied physical activity in rehabilitation facilities is manual body weight-supported treadmill training (BWSTT) (Barbeau, 2003; Dietz and Harkema, 2004). However, only a small number of studies discuss its effects on pain perception. Martin Ginis et al. reported decreases in current pain levels after single sessions of BWSTT in subjects with chronic incomplete SCI (iSCI) (Martin Ginis and Latimer, 2006). Two other studies reported improvements in health-related quality of life after BWSTT (Hicks et al., 2005; Semerjian et al., 2005) and according to Hicks et al. it might well be possible that these effects originate from decreased pain intensity (Hicks and Martin Ginis, 2008).

For severely affected patients though, BWSTT puts a substantial physical burden on therapists, who have to facilitate the desired movements of the paretic limbs. Therefore, even with the additional body-weight support system, two or three therapists are needed to train an individual with SCI. These limitations led to the development of robotic gait orthoses that allow automated moving of the legs on a treadmill (e.g. the "Lokomat", Colombo et al., 2001, see Fig. 8.1). However, to date it is unknown, whether training with such an orthosis has beneficial effects on pain, as suggested for BWSTT, or whether it even worsens pain due to the mechanical propulsion of the legs. Therefore, the aim of this study was to investigate the immediate and longitudinal effects of one month of robot assisted gait training (RAGT) on pain intensity in subjects with chronic iSCI.

8.3 Methods

8.3.1 Participants

Four women and 4 men (mean age ± SD = 58.3 ± 11.0 years) participated in this study. All had experienced an iSCI at least 12 months earlier (time since injury = 4.5 ± 4.8 years) and all suffered from pain. None of them had an orthopedic, neurological or psychiatric disease, except for the SCI. Characteristics can be found in Table 8.1. All subjects gave written informed consent and the study protocol was approved by the ethics committee of the Canton of Zurich, Switzerland. To be considered for inclusion, subjects had to be between the age of 18 and 70 with a chronic incomplete spinal cord injury (time after injury greater than 12 months). Patients had to be rated as ASIA grade C or D on the American Spinal Cord Injury Association Impairment Scale (AIS) (Marino et al., 2003). These patients are sensorimotor incomplete. While in AIS grade C patients more than half of specific key muscles below the lesion are graded a manual muscle score below 3, at least half of the muscles below the lesion in AIS D patients is graded 3 or stronger (Marino et al., 2003). The motor level of lesion should be between C4 and T11 to exclude patients with peripheral lesions. Furthermore, participants had to be unable to walk without at least moderate assistance at the time of inclusion (i.e. a score of less than 6 in the "mobility outdoors" item of the latest version of the Spinal Cord Independence Measure,

Itzkovich et al., 2007). Cognitive capacity to follow simple verbal instructions was necessary.

Exclusion criteria were similar to those as provided by the manufacturer of the Lokomat system (Hocoma AG, Volketswil, Switzerland): body weight greater than 130 kg, body height greater than 2 m, leg length difference greater than 2 cm, osteoporosis, instable fracture in lower extremity, restricted range of motion or presence of decubitus ulcer of lower extremity. Also, any of the following diseases limiting training led to exclusion of the study: arthritis causing pain while stepping; dyspnea or angina on moderate exertion; limited walking endurance due to cardiopulmonary or other diseases. Prevalence of

ID	Age (years)	Height (cm)	Weight (kg)	Sex	TSI	LL	Etiology	Pain(s)	AIS	WISCI
P01	69	178	68	m	16	C4	trauma	nbp	D	13
P02	43	163	54	w	84	T11	trauma	nap&nbp	D	12
P03	60	166	75	w	21	T4	abscess	nap&ms	D	16
P04	60	179	92	m	44	T11	hern	ms	D	9
P05	41	161	48	w	189	C6	trauma	nbp&ms	D	16
P06	53	183	85	m	29	C5	hern	nap&nbp	D	13
P07	67	164	89	w	27	C5	hern	nap&nbp	D	16
P08	69	179	93	m	26	C4	trauma	nbp&ms	D	16

Table 8.1: Characteristics of the participating patients. Abbreviations: ID = identification; TSI = time since injury in months; LL = level of lesion; AIS = ASIA Impairment Scale grade; WISCI = Walking Index for Spinal Cord Injury; C = cervical; T = thoracic; hern = herniation; nbp = neuropathic below level pain; nap = neuropathic at level pain; ms = musculoskeletal pain.

other neurological or orthopedic injuries and medical diseases which may limit exercise participation or impair locomotion (e.g. serious infection; severe orthostatic hypotension or uncontrolled hypertension, congestive heart failure, pain while weight-bearing) as well as severe metabolic diseases, epilepsy, pre-morbid ongoing major depression or psychosis were additional exclusion criteria. Patients were asked to maintain their regular medication scheme and inform the principal investigator about any changes or extraordinary events.

8.3.2 Rehabilitation device and training protocol
In this study, patient-cooperative control strategies were implemented within the Lokomat system (Figure 8.1) for RAGT. More detailed information about the Lokomat system can be found in related publications (Colombo et al., 2000; Riener et al., 2010). Briefly summarized, the Lokomat comprises two actuated leg orthoses that are attached to the patient's legs. Passive foot lifters can be added to induce ankle dorsiflexion during swing phase. Patients are connected via a harness to a bodyweight support system. This allows relieving a definable amount of the patient's weight on the legs and therefore makes performing leg movements easier. To adapt the RAGT to the patient's level of impairment we implemented 3 training modes with increasing difficulty: (i) standard mode with position control as described in (Colombo et al., 2000), (ii) interactive mode, allowing the patient to interact with the robot and adjust the walking pattern, (iii) interactive mode, allowing the patient to interact with the robot and the treadmill speed (the

interactive mode is based on path control rather than position control, see Vallery et al., 2009a,b for more information).

The patients trained for 45 min (actual training time) four times a week during a period of four weeks, i.e. each patient performed 16 training sessions in total. The first session focused on adjusting the system to the patient. To allow patients to familiarize with the system, training started with approximately 30% body-weight support and a treadmill speed between 1 and 2 km/h. All patients initially started training using foot lifters to ensure foot clearance during swing phase thereby preventing stumbling. If control and strength of ankle dorsiflexion improved, the tension of the foot lifters was decreased until volitional dorsiflexion was sufficient to remove the foot lifters. In subsequent sessions, training intensity was

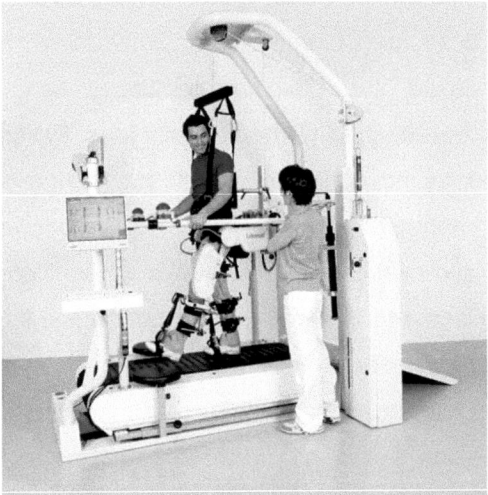

Figure 8.1: The Lokomat system (Photo courtesy of Hocoma AG)

increased progressively by changing walking speed, level of body-weight support, robotic support or by applying the next higher training mode. The amount of body-weight support was adjusted individually in order for the patients to achieve adequate knee extension during stance phase and toe clearance during swing phase.

8.3.3 Pain assessment

All patients participated in an extensive neurological examination and anamnesis. Before and after the training intervention, iSCI subjects participated in a structured pain interview where information about pain location (by drawing and pointing) and pain features (verbalized as adjectives according to Siddall et al., 1997) was obtained. Furthermore, the patients had to rate 3 domains of quality of life (QOL), namely their mood over the last week (from '0 = very bad' to '10 = very good'), their anxiety over the last week (from '0 = no fear at all' to '10 = very anxious'; for ease of interpretation, this score was reversed post-hoc so that higher scores indicated fewer anxiety to have a similar scoring system compared to the other two questions) and their general state of health over the last week ('1 = very bad', '2 = bad', '3 = satisfying', '4 = good', '5 = very good').

Pain classifications were performed by an experienced psychologist. To assess the influence of RAGT on general pain intensity, subjects were asked to rate their current pain immediately before and 5 min after each training session on a 100 mm visual analog scale (VAS) that was confined by the terms "no pain" on the left side and "unbearable pain" on the right side. The instructions were: "Please rate the general pain you are experiencing at this moment". We assessed the longitudinal influence of Lokomat trainings on the course of pain intensity over one month by plotting the mean before training values of the group against time over all 16 sessions. Additionally, we investigated the short-term effect of training on pain intensity by comparing the mean VAS values before and after each training session for the group and for each individual patient. To avoid the influence of circadian pain patterns, trainings were always performed on the same time of the day.

8.3.4 Statistical analysis

To evaluate the longitudinal influence of Lokomat training on pain intensity, we performed linear regression analyses of the mean VAS values before and after training. We considered a longitudinal decrease in pain intensity to be significant, when the regression coefficient was significantly smaller than zero. For the short-term effects of Lokomat training on pain intensity, we applied a two-way ANOVA for repeated measures, which was calculated using a mixed model, where the intensities of pre and post training pain were defined as fixed values. For the short-term effect of every single individual, we averaged the 16 pre training and the 16 post training pain intensities and applied a two-tailed Paired-Samples T-Test.

8.4 Results

One subject (P06, see Table 8.1) did not report pain any longer in the structured pain interview after the training intervention. Overall,

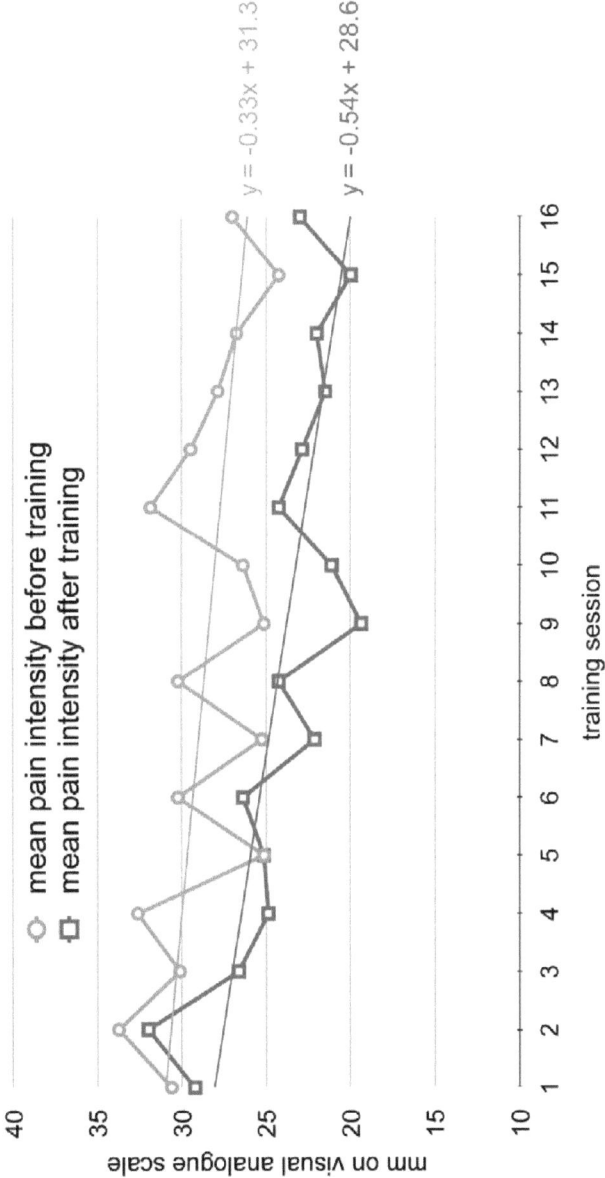

Figure 8.2: Longitudinal and short-term development of pain intensity during Lokomat training. Longitudinal change in pain

intensity before (light grey circles) and after (dark grey rectangles) robot assisted gait training in chronic incomplete spinal cord injured patients. A linear regression function was fitted through the datapoints showing that the overall decrease in pain intensity was 0.33 mm per day before training and 0.54 mm per day after training on the VAS scale. This resulted in a decrease of about 5.3 mm (before) and 8.6 mm (after) during the training period, which is about 17% and 30% of the initial values.

16 sessions of Lokomat training reduced the pain intensity over time. The slope of the mean VAS before training values (-0.33) was significantly smaller than 0 ($p = 0.04$, 95% confidence interval [CI] of the regression coefficient: [-0.05, -0.60], Figure 8.2). Also the mean VAS after training values (-0.54) showed a significant reduction of pain over time ($p = 0.01$, 95% CI: [-0.30, -0.77], Figure 8.2). With respect to the immediate influence of Lokomat training, the ANOVA for repeated measures indicated no significant difference between pre training and post training pain values ($F [1,254] = 1.69$; $p = 0.20$). If analyzed separately for each individual subject (mean VAS before training values vs. mean VAS after training values), 4 patients (P01, P03, P05, P07) showed a significant decrease, 1 (P06) a significant increase and 3 (P02, P04, P08) showed no significant differences from before to after training (Figure 8.3). There were no differences in the QOL questions from before to after the intervention (mood: before 7.38 ± 1.85 vs. after 7.50 ± 2.00, $p = 0.82$; anxiety: 8.13 ± 1.73 vs. 8.38 ± 1.77, $p = 0.63$; general state of

health: 3.25 ± 1.16 vs. 3.63 ± 1.06, p = 0.20). No training sessions had to be aborted due to pain.

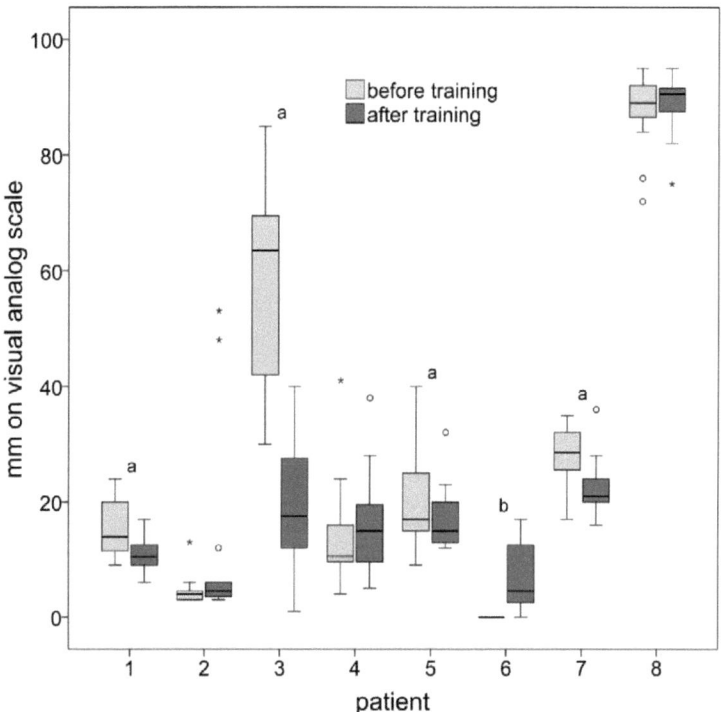

Figure 8.3: Short-term effect of Lokomat training on pain intensity for each participant. Box-plots showing the pain intensity values (median and percentiles) before (light grey) and after (dark grey) robot assisted gait training for each patient with incomplete spinal cord injury. (a) Significant (p≤0.05) decrease, and (b) significant (p≤0.05) increase in pain intensity.

8.5 Discussion

We could demonstrate for the first time that RAGT has a positive longitudinal pain-reducing effect in patients with chronic iSCI. This is in line with some sparse findings obtained from manual BWSTT studies (Hicks et al., 2005; Semerjian et al., 2005).

Overall, participants showed an alleviation of pain intensity over time, reflected in steadily decreasing VAS before and after training values. There also was a not statistically significant trend towards a reduction of pain intensity already due to single sessions of RAGT (comparison of averaged pre with post training values in Figures 8.2 and 8.3). If pain intensity was averaged over all sessions and subjects (before training: 28.6 ± 3.0 mm and after training: 24.1 ± 3.3 mm), this equaled in a mean short-term pain reduction of 15.7%, which meets the minimal clinically important difference for musculoskeletal pain (Salaffi et al., 2004). However, low sample size and high inter-subject variability (Figure 8.3) led to non-significant results in the ANOVA. Nevertheless, it can be stated that the Lokomat can be adapted to the physiology of the patients without overstraining the musculoskeletal system. In our study there was only one subject who reported a slight increase in pain intensity after the trainings compared to before, but he denied that this might have been caused by the Lokomat itself.

We did not investigate pain-relieving effects within a specific type of pain, because we had only a small number of subjects, and some of these subjects experienced both musculoskeletal and neuropathic pain. In our opinion, it might not be so relevant, as there is evidence in the literature that physical activity can have positive effects on neuropathic as well as musculoskeletal pain. Several studies suggested that physical activity could have a positive influence on impaired sensory function (Edgerton et al., 1997; Harkema et al., 1997; Hesse et al., 1995; Trimble et al., 1998) and it has been shown in animals that treadmill running has positive effects on nerve regeneration and functional recovery after peripheral nerve injuries (Marqueste et al., 2005; Sabatier et al., 2008), which are known to cause neuropathic pain (Bridges et al., 2001). Furthermore, with respect to musculoskeletal pain, literature shows that physical activity can reduce pain (Feine and Lund, 1997; Liddle et al., 2004; Mannerkorpi and Henriksson, 2007).

8.5.1 Mechanisms

The mechanisms that lead to pain relief after Lokomat training are not very well understood, especially the longitudinal effects. There are however some animal studies that address the improvement of sensory function after treadmill training (Hutchinson et al., 2004). It has been shown to affect the production of neurotrophins (e.g. brain-derived neurotrophic factor [BDNF]) in the spinal cord and skeletal muscle (Gomez-Pinilla et al., 2002). BDNF modulates sensory input within the spinal cord (Kerr et al., 1999) and it is required for tactile discrimination by slow adapting mechanoreceptors (Carroll et al., 1998). The beneficial effects of exercise and neurotrophins on sensory recovery are likely to rely on activity-dependent events within selected circuits activated by particular patterns of movements (Hutchinson et al., 2004). In treadmill locomotion the crucial afferent inputs are given by the load application on the limbs and the forced hip extension by the backward moving belt (Dietz et al., 2002). Also rhythmicity is thought to enhance sensory processing after SCI (Skinner et al., 1996). However, the influence of exercise and neurotrophins on pain intensity after SCI in humans has to be investigated more precisely.

8.5.2 Limitations

A major limitation is the study's sample size. Sample sizes are known to be rather small in exercise training studies involving people with SCI (Martin Ginis and Hicks, 2005). A greater number of participants would have allowed for greater statistical power for detecting changes in the pain measures. However, since we already got significant results, this might point out the considerable potential of this kind of rehabilitation training in the field of pain management after SCI. A second limitation is the generalizability of our findings that is limited to people with the narrowly defined inclusion and exclusion criteria applied in this study. In addition, the average intensity of pain in this sample varied much and it remains speculative whether RAGT could alleviate pain more in patients who experience weaker or in those with stronger pain. While one patient in our study with strong pain profited from the training (P03), the patient who reported the highest pain intensity (P08) did not show any change in pain intensity due to the training (see Figure 8.3).

8.6 Conclusion

In summary, the present data indicates that RAGT with the Lokomat system has a positive effect on the perceived pain intensity. This applies especially to longitudinal effects over several training sessions.

8.7 Acknowledgement

We would like to thank Alex Duschau-Wicke, PhD, for providing us with the software for the interactive training modes described in the methods section and Alex Schück for his help with the conduction of the trainings. Furthermore, we are grateful for the support of Petra Dokladal, PhD, with the pain questionnaires. Finally, we want to acknowledge the financial support of the International Spinal Research Trust (Clinical Initiative Stage 2, London, Great Britain – CLI06) and the EMDO Foundation (Zurich, Switzerland).

9 General Discussion

The general aim of this book was to provide an overview of existing outcome measures of motor function, to evaluate the newly developed assessment tools FET and RET and to test their performance and that of other outcome measures in a training intervention with iSCI patients. This led to a total of 6 studies and 1 review. The *review* delivers recommendations on which outcome measures should be used by default in the assessment of motor function after SCI and it reports that an early rehabilitation leads to better outcome compared to late rehabilitation. The *first study* investigated, whether 10MWT could be improved by implementing curves and additional tasks. The *second study* explored response time behavior of patients with SCI and presented psychometric properties of the RET. The *third study* extended these investigations to well-rehabilitated patients with iSCI and analyzed the physiological loci of the remaining deficits using TMS and EMG. The *fourth study* compared the effects of a task-specific versus task-unspecific locomotor training intervention on walking-related outcome measures in ambulating patients with iSCI. The *fifth study* looked at MEP latencies and response times in the course of these training interventions and the *sixth study* investigated the effects of RAGT on the perception of pain intensity. The findings of each individual study have been discussed in the specific discussion sections. In the following, the findings are discussed in the conjunction with each other and briefly summarized in the context of respective research questions stated in the general introduction of this book.

The review listed the currently most validated and widely spread outcome measures of motor function in the field of SCI and recommended the use of the ASIA motor score, the SCIM III and a combination of 10MWT and WISCI II. These measures have shown to be valid and reliable for the SCI population, they have been widely adopted throughout the world, enabling the comparison of data between centers, and they can be easily undertaken with a minimum of equipment. Nevertheless, there are some limitations that need to be discussed. The ASIA motor score, the SCIM and the WISCI are nonlinear ordinal scales and prone to ceiling effects in subjects with mild iSCI. The ASIA motor score has deficits specifically in the upper band of strength, as the range between a score of 3 (against gravity) and 5 (against full resistance) is much broader compared to the range between a score of 1 (palpable or visible contraction) and 3, leading to an insufficient sensitivity (Herbison et al. 1996; Noreau and Vachon 1998). The SCIM needs further refinements and psychometric validation (Anderson et al., 2008) so that it might be implemented world wide by standard (especially in the United States, where regulatory authorities still insist on the use of the FIM). These limitations confirm the need for additional functional tests, especially for AIS grade C and D patients.

This gains additional importance if it is put in the framework of regeneration-inducing therapies that are currently being developed.

Someday these therapies will hopefully also be available for subjects with mild iSCI and to test the efficacy of these treatments, outcome measures with higher sensitivity will be needed.

One such outcome measure could be response time, as it offers insights in the content, duration, and temporal course of cognitive actions combined with the execution of fast and precise movements. It includes quantification of cognitive vigilance, spinal conductivity and muscle function. With respect to adaptive ambulatory function, more sensitive tests could include higher environmental demands or dual tasking.

Chapters 3 to 7 elaborate on these outcome measures. We showed that the FET as well as the RET can be validly performed in the iSCI population. We furthermore established normative values for patients with iSCI as well as healthy controls and could demonstrate possible benefits of applying these two tests.

9.1 Figure of Eight Test

As discussed in chapter 3, we developed the FET to test the subjects' ability to adapt their gait to several circumstances and tested the ability of the different conditions to explain the variance of several established functional ambulation-related measures. Results showed higher prediction capabilities of the normal 10MWT compared to the FET conditions. We therefore suggested that the 10MWT performs better in estimating functional ambulation performance and does not need to be improved. However, as our reference measures (SCIM, FES-I, LEMS, SOT and WISCI) are potentially prone to ceiling effects, the potential use of the FET to detect differences in well-rehabilitated patients remains unclear and should be further investigated. In chapter 6 it was demonstrated that certain conditions of the FET significantly improve after a strength training intervention, whereas they did not after robotic-assisted treadmill training. In summary, the FET is a valid tool to assess adaptive walking and it adds information to the gold standard, the 10MWT.

9.2 Reaction and Execution Test

In chapter 4, validity of the RET was demonstrated for the ambulatory iSCI population. Furthermore, there were clear differences in reaction and movement time in subjects with iSCI compared to healthy controls. In the subsequent study (chapter 5), we extended the measurement by combining a set of relatively simple tests and could thusly determine different loci of interest (cortical time, conduction time, motor time, and movement time). We applied this approach to a homogenous group of well-rehabilitated iSCI patients and compared to healthy controls, we found differences in conduction and movement times, whereas there were no differences in strength of certain leg muscles. This points out the sensitivity of this method. However, we could not detect differences after the performed training interventions with the RET (chapter 7). In general, there can be two reasons for this: (1) There were no improvements in response time after the interventions. (2) The RET could not detect achieved improvements. Since we could detect already small systematic differences between healthy and patients, who recovered extremely well in chapter 5, we assume that our training interventions did not lead to improvements in response time. It thereby must be noted that the quick execution of a precise movements was not specifically trained in either intervention. In summary, the RET (especially in combination with EMG and TMS) is suggested to be useful for detecting subclinical deficits in people with mild motor impairments. The use of the RET should therefore be evaluated for other movement disorders as well.

This book extends the knowledge of motor function after spinal cord injury. The RET can be used to characterize remaining motor deficits to a higher extent compared to established measures. The FET gives additional information about the walking capacity of people with iSCI. With respect to rehabilitation, the current gait-specific rehabilitation approach should be expanded to curve-walking and complemented by strength training. To evaluate the effectiveness of upcoming regeneration-inducing therapies after incomplete spinal cord injury, it is crucial to improve the sensitivity of current clinical assessment batteries by introducing additional outcome measures, such as those presented in this work.

10 References

Ackery A, Tator C, Krassioukov A. A global perspective on spinal cord injury epidemiology. J Neurotrauma. 2004;21(10):1355-70.

Aito S, D'Andrea M, Werhagen L, Farsetti L, Cappelli S, Bandini B, et al. Neurological and functional outcome in traumatic central cord syndrome. Spinal Cord. 2007;45(4):292-7.

Alexander MS, Anderson KD, Biering-Sorensen F, Blight AR, Brannon R, Bryce TN, et al. Outcome measures in spinal cord injury: recent assessments and recommendations for future directions. Spinal Cord. 2009;47(8):582-91.

Amsters DI, Pershouse KJ, Price GL, Kendall MB. Long duration spinal cord injury: perceptions of functional change over time. Disabil Rehabil. 2005;27(9):489-97.

Anacker SL, Di Fabio RP. Influence of sensory inputs on standing balance in community-dwelling elders with a recent history of falling. Phys Ther. 1992;72(8):575-81; discussion 81-4.

Andersen JL, Mohr T, Biering-Sorensen F, Galbo H, Kjaer M. Myosin heavy chain isoform transformation in single fibers from m. vastus lateralis in spinal cord injured individuals: effects of long-term functional electrical stimulation (FES). Pflugers Arch. 1996;431(4):513-8.

Anderson KD. Targeting recovery: priorities of the spinal cord-injured population. J Neurotrauma. 2004;21(10):1371-83.

Bach M. [The Freiburg Vision Test. Automated determination of visual acuity]. Ophthalmologe. 1995;92(2):174-8.

Ballanger B, Boulinguez P. EMG as a key tool to assess motor lateralization and hand reaction time asymmetries. J Neurosci Methods. 2009;179(1):85-9.

Barbeau H. Locomotor training in neurorehabilitation: emerging rehabilitation concepts. Neurorehabil Neural Repair. 2003;17(1):3-11.

Barbeau H, Rossignol S. Recovery of locomotion after chronic spinalization in the adult cat. Brain Res. 1987;412(1):84-95.

Barbeau H, Visintin M. Optimal outcomes obtained with body-weight support combined with treadmill training in stroke subjects. Arch Phys Med Rehabil. 2003;84(10):1458-65.

Barbeau H, Elashoff R, Deforge D, Ditunno JF, Saulino M, Dobkin BH. Comparison of speeds used for the 15.2-meter and 6-minute walks over the year after an incomplete spinal cord injury: the SCILT Trial. Neurorehabil Neural Repair. 2007;21(4):302-6.

Bareyre FM, Kerschensteiner M, Raineteau O, Mettenleiter TC, Weinmann O, Schwab ME. The injured spinal cord spontaneously forms a new intraspinal circuit in adult rats. Nat Neurosci. 2004;7(3):269-77.

Barthelemy D, Nielsen JB. Corticospinal contribution to arm muscle activity during human walking. J Physiol. 2010;588(Pt 6):967-79.

Beaud ML, Schmidlin E, Wannier T, Freund P, Bloch J, Mir A, et al. Anti-Nogo-A antibody treatment does not prevent cell body shrinkage in the motor cortex in adult monkeys subjected to unilateral cervical cord lesion. BMC Neurosci. 2008;9:5.

Behrman AL, Harkema SJ. Locomotor training after human spinal cord injury: a series of case studies. Phys Ther. 2000;80(7):688-700.

Behrman AL, Harkema SJ. Physical rehabilitation as an agent for recovery after spinal cord injury. Phys Med Rehabil Clin N Am. 2007;18(2):183-202.

Belci M, Catley M, Husain M, Frankel HL, Davey NJ. Magnetic brain stimulation can improve clinical outcome in incomplete spinal cord injured patients. Spinal Cord. 2004;42(7):417-9.

Benedetti MG, Piperno R, Simoncini L, Bonato P, Tonini A, Giannini S. Gait abnormalities in minimally impaired multiple sclerosis patients. Mult Scler. 1999;5(5):363-8.

Beninato M, O'Kane KS, Sullivan PE. Relationship between motor FIM and muscle strength in lower cervical-level spinal cord injuries. Spinal Cord. 2004;42(9):533-40.

Berg KO, Wood-Dauphinee SL, Williams JI, Maki B. Measuring balance in the elderly: validation of an instrument. Can J Public Health. 1992;83 Suppl 2:S7-11.

Bilney B, Morris ME, Churchyard A, Chiu E, Georgiou-Karistianis N. Evidence for a disorder of locomotor timing in Huntington's disease. Mov Disord. 2005;20(1):51-7.

Bolliger M, Banz R, Dietz V, Lunenburger L. Standardized voluntary force measurement in a lower extremity rehabilitation robot. J Neuroeng Rehabil. 2008;5:23.

Boswell-Ruys CL, Sturnieks DL, Harvey LA, Sherrington C, Middleton JW, Lord SR. Validity and reliability of assessment tools for measuring unsupported sitting in people with a spinal cord injury. Arch Phys Med Rehabil. 2009;90(9):1571-7.

Botwinick J, Thompson LW. Premotor and motor components of reaction time. J Exp Psychol. 1966;71(1):9-15.

Bouyer LJ. Animal models for studying potential training strategies in persons with spinal cord injury. J Neurol Phys Ther. 2005;29(3):117-25.

Bridges D, Thompson SW, Rice AS. Mechanisms of neuropathic pain. Brit J Anaesth. 2001;87(1):12-26.

Brotherton SS, Krause JS, Nietert PJ. Falls in individuals with incomplete spinal cord injury. Spinal Cord. 2007;45(1):37-40.

Brouwer B, Ashby P. Corticospinal projections to lower limb motoneurons in man. Exp Brain Res. 1992;89(3):649-54.

Burns AS, Delparte JJ, Patrick M, Marino RJ, Ditunno JF. The reproducibility and convergent validity of the Walking Index for Spinal Cord Injury (WISCI) in chronic spinal cord injury. Neurorehabil Neural Repair. 2011;25(2):149-57.

Burns SP, Golding DG, Rolle WA, Jr., Graziani V, Ditunno JF. Recovery of ambulation in motor-incomplete tetraplegia. Arch Phys Med Rehabil. 1997;78(11):1169-72.

Cadotte DW, Fehlings MG. Spinal cord injury: a systematic review of current treatment options. Clin Orthop Relat Res. 2011;469(3):732-41.

Calancie B, Molano MR, Broton JG. Tendon reflexes for predicting movement recovery after acute spinal cord injury in humans. Clin Neurophysiol. 2004a;115(10):2350-63.

Calancie B, Molano MR, Broton JG. EMG for assessing the recovery of voluntary movement after acute spinal cord injury in man. Clin Neurophysiol. 2004b;115(8):1748-59.

Calancie B, Alexeeva N, Broton JG, Suys S, Hall A, Klose KJ. Distribution and latency of muscle responses to transcranial magnetic stimulation of motor cortex after spinal cord injury in humans. J Neurotrauma. 1999;16(1):49-67.

Carroll P, Lewin GR, Koltzenburg M, Toyka KV, Thoenen H. A role for BDNF in mechanosensation. Nat Neurosci. 1998;1(1):42-6.

Catz A, Itzkovich M, Agranov E, Ring H, Tamir A. SCIM--spinal cord independence measure: a new disability scale for patients with spinal cord lesions. Spinal Cord. 1997;35(12):850-6.

Catz A, Greenberg E, Itzkovich M, Bluvshtein V, Ronen J, Gelernter I. A new instrument for outcome assessment in rehabilitation medicine: Spinal cord injury ability realization measurement index. Arch Phys Med Rehabil. 2004;85(3):399-404.

Catz A, Itzkovich M, Steinberg F, Philo O, Ring H, Ronen J, et al. The Catz-Itzkovich SCIM: a revised version of the Spinal Cord Independence Measure. Disabil Rehabil. 2001;23(6):263-8.

Catz A, Itzkovich M, Tesio L, Biering-Sorensen F, Weeks C, Laramee MT, et al. A multicenter international study on the Spinal Cord Independence Measure, version III: Rasch psychometric validation. Spinal Cord. 2007;45(4):275-91.

Cerny D, Waters R, Hislop H, Perry J. Walking and wheelchair energetics in persons with paraplegia. Phys Ther. 1980;60(9):1133-9.

Chang JJ, Tung WL, Wu WL, Su FC. Effect of bilateral reaching on affected arm motor control in stroke--with and without loading on unaffected arm. Disabil Rehabil. 2006;28(24):1507-16.

Chapman JP, Chapman LJ, Allen JJ. The measurement of foot preference. Neuropsychologia. 1987;25(3):579-84.

Chen HC, Ashton-Miller JA, Alexander NB, Schultz AB. Effects of age and available response time on ability to step over an obstacle. J Gerontol. 1994;49(5):M227-33.

Chiou II, Burnett CN. Values of activities of daily living. A survey of stroke patients and their home therapists. Phys Ther. 1985;65(6):901-6.

Cifu DX, Seel RT, Kreutzer JS, McKinley WO. A multicenter investigation of age-related differences in lengths of stay, hospitalization charges, and outcomes for a matched tetraplegia sample. Arch Phys Med Rehabil. 1999;80(7):733-40.

Cohen J. Statistical Power Analysis for the Behavioral Sciences (2nd edition)
Lawrence Erlbaum Associates, Inc.; Hillsdale, NJ, USA. 1988.

Colombo G, Wirz M, Dietz V. Driven gait orthosis for improvement of locomotor training in paraplegic patients. Spinal Cord. 2001;39(5):252-5.

Colombo G, Joerg M, Schreier R, Dietz V. Treadmill training of paraplegic patients using a robotic orthosis. J Rehabil Res Dev. 2000;37(6):693-700.

Consortium for Spinal Cord Medicine. Outcomes following traumatic spinal cord injury: clinical practice guidelines for health-care professionals. J Spinal Cord Med. 2000;23(4):289-316.

Crameri RM, Weston A, Climstein M, Davis GM, Sutton JR. Effects of electrical stimulation-induced leg training on skeletal muscle adaptability in spinal cord injury. Scand J Med Sci Sports. 2002;12(5):316-22.

Curt A, Dietz V. Traumatic cervical spinal cord injury: relation between somatosensory evoked potentials, neurological deficit, and hand function. Arch Phys Med Rehabil. 1996a;77(1):48-53.

Curt A, Dietz V. Neurographic assessment of intramedullary motoneurone lesions in cervical spinal cord injury: consequences for hand function. Spinal Cord. 1996b;34(6):326-32.

Curt A, Dietz V. Ambulatory capacity in spinal cord injury: significance of somatosensory evoked potentials and ASIA protocol in predicting outcome. Arch Phys Med Rehabil. 1997;78(1):39-43.

Curt A, Keck ME, Dietz V. Functional outcome following spinal cord injury: significance of motor-evoked potentials and ASIA scores. Arch Phys Med Rehabil. 1998;79(1):81-6.

Curt A, Schwab ME, Dietz V. Providing the clinical basis for new interventional therapies: refined diagnosis and assessment of recovery after spinal cord injury. Spinal Cord. 2004;42(1):1-6.

Curt A, Van Hedel HJ, Klaus D, Dietz V. Recovery from a spinal cord injury: significance of compensation, neural plasticity, and repair. J Neurotrauma. 2008;25(6):677-85.

Dahlberg A, Kotila M, Kautiainen H, Alaranta H. Functional independence in persons with spinal cord injury in Helsinki. J Rehabil Med. 2003;35(5):217-20.

Dahlgren A, Karlsson AK, Lundgren-Nilsson A, Friden J, Claesson L. Activity performance and upper extremity function in cervical spinal cord injury patients according to the Klein-Bell ADL Scale. Spinal Cord. 2007;45(7):475-84.

Datta S, Lorenz DJ, Morrison S, Ardolino E, Harkema SJ. A multivariate examination of temporal changes in Berg Balance Scale items for patients with ASIA Impairment Scale C and D spinal cord injuries. Arch Phys Med Rehabil. 2009;90(7):1208-17.

Daverat P, Sibrac MC, Dartigues JF, Mazaux JM, Marit E, Debelleix X, et al. Early prognostic factors for walking in spinal cord injuries. Paraplegia. 1988;26(4):255-61.

Day BL, Rothwell JC, Thompson PD, Maertens de Noordhout A, Nakashima K, Shannon K, et al. Delay in the execution of voluntary movement by electrical or magnetic brain stimulation in intact man. Evidence for the storage of motor programs in the brain. Brain. 1989;112(Pt 3):649-63.

De Beaumont L, Theoret H, Mongeon D, Messier J, Leclerc S, Tremblay S, Ellemberg D, Lassonde M. Brain function decline in healthy retired athletes who sustained their last sports concussion in early adulthood. Brain. 2009;132(Pt 3):695-708.

De Vivo MJ, Richards JS, Stover SL, Go BK. Spinal cord injury. Rehabilitation adds life to years. West J Med. 1991;154(5):602-6.

De Vivo M, Biering-Sorensen F, Charlifue S, Noonan V, Post M, Stripling T, et al. International Spinal Cord Injury Core Data Set. Spinal Cord. 2006;44(9):535-40.

Delmonico MJ, Kostek MC, Doldo NA, Hand BD, Bailey JA, Rabon-Stith KM, et al. Effects of moderate-velocity strength training on peak muscle power and movement velocity: do women respond differently than men? J Appl Phys. 2005;99(5):1712-8.

Deng AW, Wei D, Zhang JH, Ran CF, Wang M. [Rehabilitation therapy in early stage following spinal cord injuries]. Di Yi Jun Yi Da Xue Xue Bao. 2004;24(6):706-7, 10.

Diehl P, Kliesch U, Dietz V, Curt A. Impaired facilitation of motor evoked potentials in incomplete spinal cord injury. J Neurol. 2006;253(1):51-7.

Dietz V. Spinal cord pattern generators for locomotion. Clin Neurophysiol. 2003;114(8):1379-89.

Dietz V, Harkema SJ. Locomotor activity in spinal cord-injured persons. J Appl Physiol. 2004;96(5):1954-60.

Dietz V, Muller R, Colombo G. Locomotor activity in spinal man: significance of afferent input from joint and load receptors. Brain. 2002;125(Pt 12):2626-34.

Dietz V, Colombo G, Jensen L, Baumgartner L. Locomotor capacity of spinal cord in paraplegic patients. Ann Neurol. 1995;37(5):574-82.

Ding Y, Kastin AJ, Pan W. Neural plasticity after spinal cord injury. Curr Pharm Design. 2005;11(11):1441-50.

Ditunno JF, Scivoletto G. Clinical relevance of gait research applied to clinical trials in spinal cord injury. Brain Res Bull. 2009;78(1):35-42.

Ditunno JF. Outcome measures: evolution in clinical trials of neurological / functional recovery in spinal cord injury. Spinal Cord. 2010;48(9):674-84.

Ditunno PL, Patrick M, Stineman M, Ditunno JF. Who wants to walk? Preferences for recovery after SCI: a longitudinal and cross-sectional study. Spinal Cord. 2008a;46(7):500-6.

Ditunno JF, Scivoletto G, Patrick M, Biering-Sorensen F, Abel R, Marino R. Validation of the walking index for spinal cord injury in a US and European clinical population. Spinal Cord. 2008b;46(3):181-8.

Ditunno JF, Ditunno PL, Graziani V, Scivoletto G, Bernardi M, Castellano V, et al. Walking index for spinal cord injury (WISCI): an international multicenter validity and reliability study. Spinal Cord. 2000;38(4):234-43.

Ditunno JF, Barbeau H, Dobkin BH, Elashoff R, Harkema S, Marino RJ, et al. Validity of the walking scale for spinal cord injury and other domains of function in a multicenter clinical trial. Neurorehabil Neural Repair. 2007;21(6):539-50.

Ditunno PL, Ditunno JF. Walking index for spinal cord injury (WISCI II): scale revision. Spinal Cord. 2001;39(12):654-6.

Dobkin B. An Overview of Treadmill Locomotor Training with Partial Body Weight Support: A Neurophysiologically Sound Approach Whose Time Has Come for Randomized Clinical Trials. Neurorehabil Neural Repair. 1999;13:157-65.

Dobkin B, Barbeau H, Deforge D, Ditunno JF, Elashoff R, Apple D, et al. The evolution of walking-related outcomes over the first 12 weeks of rehabilitation for incomplete traumatic spinal cord injury: the multicenter randomized Spinal Cord Injury Locomotor Trial. Neurorehabil Neural Repair. 2007;21(1):25-35.

Dunlap WP, Cortina JM, Vaslow JB, Burke MJ. Meta-Analysis of Experiments With Matched Groups or Repeated Measures Designs. Psychol Methods. 1996;1(2):170-7.

Duysens J, Van de Crommert HW. Neural control of locomotion; The central pattern generator from cats to humans. Gait Posture. 1998;7(2):131-41.

Dvorak MF, Fisher CG, Hoekema J, Boyd M, Noonan V, Wing PC, et al. Factors predicting motor recovery and functional outcome after traumatic central cord syndrome: a long-term follow-up. Spine. 2005;30(20):2303-11.

Eberhard S. Statistik der stationären Behandlung bei Querschnittlähmung in der Schweiz. Managed Care. 2004;2:8-11.

Edgerton VR, Tillakaratne NJ, Bigbee AJ, de Leon RD, Roy RR. Plasticity of the spinal neural circuitry after injury. Annu Rev Neurosci. 2004;27:145-67.

Edgerton VR, Roy RR, Allen DL, Monti RJ. Adaptations in skeletal muscle disuse or decreased-use atrophy. Am J Phys Med Rehabil. 2002;81(11 Suppl):S127-47.

Edgerton VR, de Leon RD, Tillakaratne N, Recktenwald MR, Hodgson JA, Roy RR. Use-dependent plasticity in spinal stepping and standing. Adv Neurol. 1997;72:233-47.

Eftekharpour E, Karimi-Abdolrezaee S, Wang J, El Beheiry H, Morshead C, Fehlings MG. Myelination of congenitally dysmyelinated spinal cord axons by adult neural precursor cells results in formation of nodes of Ranvier and improved axonal conduction. J Neurosci. 2007;27(13):3416-28.

Eide PK. Pathophysiological mechanisms of central neuropathic pain after spinal cord injury. Spinal Cord. 1998;36(9):601-12.

Ellaway PH, Catley M, Davey NJ, Kuppuswamy A, Strutton P, Frankel HL, et al. Review of physiological motor outcome measures in spinal cord injury using transcranial magnetic stimulation and spinal reflexes. J Rehabil Res Dev. 2007;44(1):69-76.

Feine JS, Lund JP. An assessment of the efficacy of physical therapy and physical modalities for the control of chronic musculoskeletal pain. Pain. 1997;71(1):5-23.

Field-Fote EC, Roach KE. Influence of a locomotor training approach on walking speed and distance in people with chronic spinal cord injury: a randomized clinical trial. Phys Ther. 2011;91(1):48-60.

Field-Fote EC, Lindley SD, Sherman AL. Locomotor training approaches for individuals with spinal cord injury: a preliminary report of walking-related outcomes. J Neurol Phys Ther. 2005;29(3):127-37.

Fisher CG, Noonan VK, Smith DE, Wing PC, Dvorak MF, Kwon BK. Motor recovery, functional status, and health-related quality of life in patients with complete spinal cord injuries. Spine. 2005;30(19):2200-7.

Folstein MF, Folstein SE, McHugh PR. "Mini-mental state". A practical method for grading the cognitive state of patients for the clinician. J Psychiatr Res. 1975;12(3):189-98.

Fouad K, Tetzlaff W. Rehabilitative training and plasticity following spinal cord injury. Exp Neurol. 2011. DOI: 10.1016/j.expneurol.2011.02.009 (Epub ahead of print, February 17.).

Frankel HL, Hancock DO, Hyslop G, Melzak J, Michaelis LS, Ungar GH, et al. The value of postural reduction in the initial management of closed injuries of the spine with paraplegia and tetraplegia. Paraplegia. 1969;7(3):179-92.

Frankel HL, Coll JR, Charlifue SW, Whiteneck GG, Gardner BP, Jamous MA, et al. Long-term survival in spinal cord injury: a fifty year investigation. Spinal Cord. 1998;36(4):266-74.

Freund P, Weiskopf N, Ward NS, Hutton C, Gall A, Ciccarelli O, et al. Disability, atrophy and cortical reorganization following spinal cord injury. Brain. 2011;134(Pt 6):1610-22.

Furlan JC, Noonan V, Singh A, Fehlings M. Assessment of disability in patients with acute traumatic spinal cord injury: A systematic review of the literature. J Neurotrauma. 2011;28(8):1413-30.

Gabbard C, Hart S. A question of foot dominance. J Gen Psychol. 1996;123(4):289-96.

Gomez-Pinilla F, Ying Z, Roy RR, Molteni R, Edgerton VR. Voluntary exercise induces a BDNF-mediated mechanism that promotes neuroplasticity. J Neurophysiol. 2002;88(5):2187-95.

Gorassini MA, Norton JA, Nevett-Duchcherer J, Roy FD, Yang JF. Changes in locomotor muscle activity after treadmill training in subjects with incomplete spinal cord injury. J Neurophysiol. 2009;101(2):969-79.

Granat MH, Ferguson AC, Andrews BJ, Delargy M. The role of functional electrical stimulation in the rehabilitation of patients with incomplete spinal cord injury--observed benefits during gait studies. Paraplegia. 1993;31(4):207-15.

Green JB, Sora E, Bialy Y, Ricamato A, Thatcher RW. Cortical motor reorganization after paraplegia: an EEG study. Neurology. 1999;53(4):736-43.

Greenwald BD, Seel RT, Cifu DX, Shah AN. Gender-related differences in acute rehabilitation lengths of stay, charges, and functional outcomes for a matched sample with spinal cord injury: a multicenter investigation. Arch Phys Med Rehabil. 2001;82(9):1181-7.

Gregory CM, Bowden MG, Jayaraman A, Shah P, Behrman A, Kautz SA, et al. Resistance training and locomotor recovery after incomplete spinal cord injury: a case series. Spinal Cord. 2007;45(7):522-30.

Grillner S. The spinal locomotor CPG: a target after spinal cord injury. Prog Brain Res. 2002;137:97-108.

Guglielmetti S, Nardone A, De Nunzio AM, Godi M, Schieppati M. Walking along circular trajectories in Parkinson's disease. Mov Disord. 2009;24(4):598-604.

Haisma JA, Post MW, van der Woude LH, Stam HJ, Bergen MP, Sluis TA, et al. Functional independence and health-related functional status following spinal cord injury: a prospective study of the association with physical capacity. J Rehabil Med. 2008;40(10):812-8.

Harada ND, Chiu V, Stewart AL. Mobility-related function in older adults: assessment with a 6-minute walk test. Arch Phys Med Rehabil. 1999;80(7):837-41.

Harkema SJ. Neural plasticity after human spinal cord injury: application of locomotor training to the rehabilitation of walking. Neuroscientist. 2001;7(5):455-68.

Harkema SJ, Hurley SL, Patel UK, Requejo PS, Dobkin BH, Edgerton VR. Human lumbosacral spinal cord interprets loading during stepping. J Neurophysiol. 1997;77(2):797-811.

Harness ET, Yozbatiran N, Cramer SC. Effects of intense exercise in chronic spinal cord injury. Spinal Cord. 2008;46(11):733-7.

Harvey LA, Batty J, Fahey A. Reliability of a tool for assessing mobility in wheelchair-dependent paraplegics. Spinal Cord. 1998;36(6):427-31.

Herbison GJ, Isaac Z, Cohen ME, Ditunno JF. Strength post-spinal cord injury: myometer vs manual muscle test. Spinal Cord. 1996;34(9):543-8.

Hess JA, Woollacott M. Effect of high-intensity strength-training on functional measures of balance ability in balance-impaired older adults. J Manip Phys Ther. 2005;28(8):582-90.

Hess RJ, Brach JS, Piva SR, Vanswearingen JM. Walking Skill Can Be Assessed in Older Adults: Validity of the Figure-of-8 Walk Test. Phys Ther. 2009;90(1):89-99.

Hesse S, Schmidt H, Werner C, Bardeleben A. Upper and lower extremity robotic devices for rehabilitation and for studying motor control. Curr Opin Neurol. 2003;16(6):705-10.

Hesse S, Bertelt C, Schaffrin A, Malezic M, Mauritz KH. Restoration of gait in nonambulatory hemiparetic patients by treadmill training with partial body-weight support. Arch Phys Med Rehabil. 1994;75(10):1087-93.

Hesse S, Bertelt C, Jahnke MT, Schaffrin A, Baake P, Malezic M, et al. Treadmill training with partial body weight support compared with physiotherapy in nonambulatory hemiparetic patients. Stroke. 1995;26(6):976-81.

Heutink M, Post MW, Wollaars MM, van Asbeck FW. Chronic spinal cord injury pain: pharmacological and non-pharmacological treatments and treatment effectiveness. Disabil Rehabil. 2011;33(5):433-40.

Hicks AL, Martin Ginis KA. Treadmill training after spinal cord injury: it's not just about the walking. J Rehabil Res Dev. 2008;45(2):241-8.

Hicks AL, Adams MM, Martin Ginis KA, Giangregorio L, Latimer A, Phillips SM, et al. Long-term body-weight-supported treadmill training and subsequent follow-up in persons with chronic SCI: effects on functional walking ability and measures of subjective well-being. Spinal Cord. 2005;43(5):291-8.

Hidler J, Nichols D, Pelliccio M, Brady K, Campbell DD, Kahn JH, et al. Multicenter randomized clinical trial evaluating the effectiveness of the lokomat in subacute stroke. Neurorehabil Neural Repair. 2009;23(1):5-13.

Hill MR, Noonan VK, Sakakibara BM, Miller WC. Quality of life instruments and definitions in individuals with spinal cord injury: a systematic review. Spinal Cord. 2010;48(6):438-50.

Hol AT, Eng JJ, Miller WC, Sproule S, Krassioukov AV. Reliability and validity of the six-minute arm test for the evaluation of cardiovascular fitness in people with spinal cord injury. Arch Phys Med Rehabil. 2007;88(4):489-95.

Hornby TG, Campbell DD, Kahn JH, Demott T, Moore JL, Roth HR. Enhanced gait-related improvements after therapist- versus robotic-assisted locomotor training in subjects with chronic stroke: a randomized controlled study. Stroke. 2008;39(6):1786-92.

Houle JD, Tessler A. Repair of chronic spinal cord injury. Exp Neurol. 2003;182(2):247-60.

Hutchinson KJ, Gomez-Pinilla F, Crowe MJ, Ying Z, Basso DM. Three exercise paradigms differentially improve sensory recovery after spinal cord contusion in rats. Brain. 2004;127(Pt 6):1403-14.

Huxham FE, Goldie PA, Patla AE. Theoretical considerations in balance assessment. Aust J Physiother. 2001;47(2):89-100.

Hyndman D, Ashburn A, Stack E. Fall events among people with stroke living in the community: circumstances of falls and characteristics of fallers. Arch Phys Med Rehabil. 2002;83(2):165-70.

IJzerman MJ, Baardman G, van 't Hof MA, Boom HB, Hermens HJ, Veltink PH. Validity and reproducibility of crutch force and heart rate measurements to assess energy expenditure of paraplegic gait. Arch Phys Med Rehabil. 1999;80(9):1017-23.

Itzkovich M, Tripolski M, Zeilig G, Ring H, Rosentul N, Ronen J, et al. Rasch analysis of the Catz-Itzkovich spinal cord independence measure. Spinal Cord. 2002;40(8):396-407.

Itzkovich M, Tamir A, Philo O, Steinberg F, Ronen J, Spasser R, et al. Reliability of the Catz-Itzkovich Spinal Cord Independence Measure assessment by interview and comparison with observation. Am J Phys Med Rehabil. 2003;82(4):267-72.

Itzkovich M, Gelernter I, Biering-Sorensen F, Weeks C, Laramee MT, Craven BC, et al. The Spinal Cord Independence Measure (SCIM) version III: reliability and validity in a multi-center international study. Disabil Rehabil. 2007;29(24):1926-33.

Jackson AB, Carnel CT, Ditunno JF, Read MS, Boninger ML, Schmeler MR, et al. Outcome measures for gait and ambulation in the spinal cord injury population. J Spinal Cord Med. 2008;31(5):487-99.

Jacobs PL, Mahoney ET, Johnson B. Reliability of arm Wingate Anaerobic Testing in persons with complete paraplegia. J Spinal Cord Med. 2003;26(2):141-4.

Jacquemin GL, Burns SP, Little JW. Measuring hand intrinsic muscle strength: normal values and interrater reliability. J Spinal Cord Med. 2004;27(5):460-7.

Jayaraman A, Gregory CM, Bowden M, Stevens JE, Shah P, Behrman AL, et al. Lower extremity skeletal muscle function in persons with incomplete spinal cord injury. Spinal Cord. 2006;44(11):680-7.

Jayaraman A, Shah P, Gregory C, Bowden M, Stevens J, Bishop M, et al. Locomotor training and muscle function after incomplete spinal cord injury: case series. J Spinal Cord Med. 2008;31(2):185-93.

Jeffery DT, Norton JA, Roy FD, Gorassini MA. Effects of transcranial direct current stimulation on the excitability of the leg motor cortex. Exp Brain Res. 2007;182(2):281-7.

Jurkiewicz MT, Mikulis DJ, McIlroy WE, Fehlings MG, Verrier MC. Sensorimotor cortical plasticity during recovery following spinal cord injury: a longitudinal fMRI study. Neurorehabil Neural Repair. 2007;21(6):527-38.

Kerr BJ, Bradbury EJ, Bennett DL, Trivedi PM, Dassan P, French J, et al. Brain-derived neurotrophic factor modulates nociceptive sensory inputs and NMDA-evoked responses in the rat spinal cord. J Neurosci. 1999;19(12):5138-48.

Kilkens OJ, Dallmeijer AJ, De Witte LP, Van Der Woude LH, Post MW. The Wheelchair Circuit: Construct validity and responsiveness of a test to assess manual wheelchair mobility in persons with spinal cord injury. Arch Phys Med Rehabil. 2004;85(3):424-31.

Kim CM, Eng JJ, Whittaker MW. Level walking and ambulatory capacity in persons with incomplete spinal cord injury: relationship with muscle strength. Spinal Cord. 2004;42(3):156-62.

Kim MO, Burns AS, Ditunno JF, Marino RJ. The assessment of walking capacity using the walking index for spinal cord injury: self-selected versus maximal levels. Arch Phys Med Rehabil. 2007;88(6):762-7.

King LA, St George RJ, Carlson-Kuhta P, Nutt JG, Horak FB. Preparation for compensatory forward stepping in Parkinson's disease. Arch Phys Med Rehabil. 2010;91(9):1332-8.

Kirby RL, Swuste J, Dupuis DJ, MacLeod DA, Monroe R. The Wheelchair Skills Test: a pilot study of a new outcome measure. Arch Phys Med Rehabil. 2002;83(1):10-8.

Kirshblum S, Millis S, McKinley W, Tulsky D. Late neurologic recovery after traumatic spinal cord injury. Arch Phys Med Rehabil. 2004;85(11):1811-7.

Kokotilo KJ, Eng JJ, Curt A. Reorganization and preservation of motor control of the brain in spinal cord injury: a systematic review. J Neurotrauma. 2009;26(11):2113-26.

Krawetz P, Nance P. Gait analysis of spinal cord injured subjects: effects of injury level and spasticity. Arch Phys Med Rehabil. 1996;77(7):635-8.

Kuper M, Brandauer B, Thurling M, Schoch B, Gizewski ER, Timmann D, Hermsdorfer J. Impaired prehension is associated with lesions of the superior and inferior hand representation within the human cerebellum. J Neurophysiol. 2011;105(5):2018-29.

Kuppuswamy A, Balasubramaniam AV, Maksimovic R, Mathias CJ, Gall A, Craggs MD, et al. Action of 5Hz repetitive transcranial magnetic stimulation on sensory, motor and autonomic function in human spinal cord injury. Clin Neurophysiol. 2011. DOI: 10.1016/j.clinph.2011.04.022 (Epub ahead of print, May 19.).

Kwon BK, Okon E, Hillyer J, Mann C, Baptiste D, Weaver LC, et al. A Systematic Review of Non-Invasive Pharmacologic Neuroprotective Treatments for Acute Spinal Cord Injury. J Neurotrauma. 2011a;28(8):1545-88.

Kwon BK, Okon EB, Plunet W, Baptiste D, Fouad K, Hillyer J, et al. A Systematic Review of Directly Applied Biologic Therapies for Acute Spinal Cord Injury. J Neurotrauma. 2011b;28(8):1589-610.

Labruyère R, van Hedel H. Instrument validity and reliability of a choice response time test for incomplete spinal cord injured subjects: relationship with function. Arch Phys Med Rehabil. 2011;92(9):1443-9

Labruyère R, Agarwala A, Curt A. Rehabilitation in spine and spinal cord trauma. Spine. 2010;35(21 Suppl):S259-62.

Ladouceur M, Barbeau H, McFadyen BJ. Kinematic adaptations of spinal cord-injured subjects during obstructed walking. Neurorehabil Neural Repair. 2003;17(1):25-31.

Lajoie Y, Barbeau H, Hamelin M. Attentional requirements of walking in spinal cord injured patients compared to normal subjects. Spinal Cord. 1999;37(4):245-50.

Lam T, Noonan VK, Eng JJ. A systematic review of functional ambulation outcome measures in spinal cord injury. Spinal Cord. 2008;46(4):246-54.

Lapointe R, Lajoie Y, Serresse O, Barbeau H. Functional community ambulation requirements in incomplete spinal cord injured subjects. Spinal Cord. 2001;39(6):327-35.

Laufer Y, Dickstein R, Chefez Y, Marcovitz E. The effect of treadmill training on the ambulation of stroke survivors in the early stages of rehabilitation: a randomized study. J Rehabil Res Dev. 2001;38(1):69-78.

Lawton G, Lundgren-Nilsson A, Biering-Sorensen F, Tesio L, Slade A, Penta M, et al. Cross-cultural validity of FIM in spinal cord injury. Spinal Cord. 2006;44(12):746-52.

Lazar RB, Yarkony GM, Ortolano D, Heinemann AW, Perlow E, Lovell L, et al. Prediction of functional outcome by motor capability after spinal cord injury. Arch Phys Med Rehabil. 1989;70(12):819-22.

Leocani L, Cohen LG, Wassermann EM, Ikoma K, Hallett M. Human corticospinal excitability evaluated with transcranial magnetic stimulation during different reaction time paradigms. Brain. 2000;123 (Pt 6):1161-73.

Liddle SD, Baxter GD, Gracey JH. Exercise and chronic low back pain: what works? Pain. 2004;107(1-2):176-90.

Lim HK, Lee DC, McKay WB, Priebe MM, Holmes SA, Sherwood AM. Neurophysiological assessment of lower-limb voluntary control in incomplete spinal cord injury. Spinal Cord. 2005;43(5):283-90.

Lim HK, Lee DC, McKay WB, Protas EJ, Holmes SA, Priebe MM, et al. Analysis of sEMG during voluntary movement--Part II: Voluntary response index sensitivity. IEEE T Neur Sys Rehabil. 2004;12(4):416-21.

Lings S. Assessing driving capability: a method for individual testing: the significance of paraparesis inferior studied in a controlled experiment. Appl Ergon. 1991;22(2):75-84.

Lord SR, Clark RD. Simple physiological and clinical tests for the accurate prediction of falling in older people. Gerontology. 1996;42(4):199-203.

Lord SR, Fitzpatrick RC. Choice stepping reaction time: a composite measure of falls risk in older people. J Gerontol A Biol Sci Med Sci. 2001;56(10):M627-32.

Lord SR, Clark RD, Webster IW. Postural stability and associated physiological factors in a population of aged persons. J Gerontol. 1991;46(3):M69-76.

Lynch SM, Leahy P, Barker SP. Reliability of measurements obtained with a modified functional reach test in subjects with spinal cord injury. Phys Ther. 1998;78(2):128-33.

Mace SE, Brown LA, Francis L, Godwin SA, Hahn SA, Howard PK, et al. Clinical policy: Critical issues in the sedation of pediatric patients in the emergency department. Ann Emerg Med. 2008;51(4):378-99, 99 e1-57.

Maki BE, McIlroy WE. The role of limb movements in maintaining upright stance: the "change-in-support" strategy. Phys Ther. 1997;77(5):488-507.

Maki BE, Holliday PJ, Topper AK. A prospective study of postural balance and risk of falling in an ambulatory and independent elderly population. J Gerontol. 1994;49(2):M72-84.

Mannerkorpi K, Henriksson C. Non-pharmacological treatment of chronic widespread musculoskeletal pain. Best Pract Res Cl RH. 2007;21(3):513-34.

Marcotte TD, Rosenthal TJ, Roberts E, Lampinen S, Scott JC, Allen RW, et al. The contribution of cognition and spasticity to driving performance in multiple sclerosis. Arch Phys Med Rehabil. 2008;89(9):1753-8.

Marino RJ, Graves DE. Metric properties of the ASIA motor score: subscales improve correlation with functional activities. Arch Phys Med Rehabil 2004;85(11):1804-10.

Marino RJ, Shea JA, Stineman MG. The Capabilities of Upper Extremity instrument: reliability and validity of a measure of functional limitation in tetraplegia. Arch Phys Med Rehabil. 1998;79(12):1512-21.

Marino RJ, Herbison GJ, Ditunno JF. Peripheral sprouting as a mechanism for recovery in the zone of injury in acute quadriplegia: A single fiber EMG study. Muscle Nerve. 1994;17(12):1466-8.

Marino RJ, Ditunno JF, Donovan WH, Maynard F, Jr. Neurologic recovery after traumatic spinal cord injury: data from the Model Spinal Cord Injury Systems. Arch Phys Med Rehabil. 1999;80(11):1391-6.

Marino RJ, Barros T, Biering-Sorensen F, Burns SP, Donovan WH, Graves DE, et al. International standards for neurological classification of spinal cord injury. J Spinal Cord Med. 2003;26 Suppl 1:S50-6.

Marqueste T, Alliez JR, Alluin O, Jammes Y, Decherchi P. Neuromuscular rehabilitation by treadmill running or electrical stimulation after peripheral nerve injury and repair. J Appl Physiol. 2004;96(5):1988-95.

Martin Ginis KA, Hicks AL. Exercise research issues in the spinal cord injured population. Exerc Sport Sci Rev. 2005;33(1):49-53.

Martin Ginis KA, Latimer AE. The effects of single bouts of body-weight supported treadmill training on the feeling states of people with spinal cord injury. Spinal Cord. 2007;45(1):112-5.

Martin Ginis KA, Latimer AE, McKechnie K, Ditor DS, McCartney N, Hicks AL, et al. Using exercise to enhance subjective well-being among people with incomplete spinal cord injury: The mediating influences of stress and pain. Rehabil Psychol. 2003;48(3):157-64.

May LA, Butt C, Minor L, Kolbinson K, Tulloch K. Measurement reliability of functional tasks for persons who self-propel a manual wheelchair. Arch Phys Med Rehabil. 2003;84(4):578-83.

Mayr A, Kofler M, Quirbach E, Matzak H, Frohlich K, Saltuari L. Prospective, blinded, randomized crossover study of gait rehabilitation in stroke patients using the Lokomat gait orthosis. Neurorehabil Neural Repair. 2007;21(4):307-14.

Mazzucchi A, Sinforiani E, Ludovico L, Turla M, Pacchetti C, Brianti R, et al. Reaction time responses in parkinsonian and hemiparkinsonian patients. Mov Disord. 1993;8(1):13-8.

McKinley W, Santos K, Meade M, Brooke K. Incidence and outcomes of spinal cord injury clinical syndromes. J Spinal Cord Med. 2007;30(3):215-24.

Mehrholz J, Kugler J, Pohl M. Locomotor training for walking after spinal cord injury. Cochrane Database Syst Rev. 2008(2):CD006676.

Melis EH, Torres-Moreno R, Barbeau H, Lemaire ED. Analysis of assisted-gait characteristics in persons with incomplete spinal cord injury. Spinal Cord. 1999;37(6):430-9.

Melzer I, Tzedek I, Or M, Shvarth G, Nizri O, Ben-Shitrit K, et al. Speed of voluntary stepping in chronic stroke survivors under single- and dual-task conditions: a case-control study. Arch Phys Med Rehabil. 2009;90(6):927-33.

Metter EJ, Schrager M, Ferrucci L, Talbot LA. Evaluation of movement speed and reaction time as predictors of all-cause mortality in men. J Gerontol A Biol Sci Med Sci. 2005;60(7):840-6.

Middleton JW, Harvey LA, Batty J, Cameron I, Quirk R, Winstanley J. Five additional mobility and locomotor items to improve responsiveness of the FIM in wheelchair-dependent individuals with spinal cord injury. Spinal Cord. 2006;44(8):495-504.

Miller J. A warning about median reaction time. J Exp Psychol Hum Percept Perform. 1988;14(3):539-43.

Morganti B, Scivoletto G, Ditunno P, Ditunno JF, Molinari M. Walking index for spinal cord injury (WISCI): criterion validation. Spinal Cord. 2005;43(1):27-33.

Mulcahey MJ, Hutchinson D, Kozin S. Assessment of upper limb in tetraplegia: considerations in evaluation and outcomes research. J Rehabil Res Dev. 2007;44(1):91-102.

Musselman K, Brunton K, Lam T, Yang J. Spinal cord injury functional ambulation profile: a new measure of walking ability. Neurorehabil Neural Repair. 2011;25(3):285-93.

Musselman KE, Yang JF. Walking tasks encountered by urban-dwelling adults and persons with incomplete spinal cord injuries. J Rehabil Med. 2007;39(7):567-74.

National Spinal Cord Injury Statistical Center. Fact and Figures 2010. https://www.nscisc.uab.edu. Accessed March 27, 2010.

National Spinal Cord Injury Statistical Center. Fact and Figures 2011. https://www.nscisc.uab.edu. Accessed September 4, 2011.

Nepomuceno C, Fine PR, Richards JS, Gowens H, Stover SL, Rantanuabol U, et al. Pain in patients with spinal cord injury. Arch Phys Med Rehabil. 1979;60(12):605-9.

Nooijen CF, Ter Hoeve N, Field-Fote EC. Gait quality is improved by locomotor training in individuals with SCI regardless of training approach. J Neuroeng Rehabil. 2009;6:36.

Noreau L, Vachon J. Comparison of three methods to assess muscular strength in individuals with spinal cord injury. Spinal Cord. 1998;36(10):716-23.

Norton JA, Gorassini MA. Changes in cortically related intermuscular coherence accompanying improvements in locomotor skills in incomplete spinal cord injury. J Neurophysiol. 2006;95(4):2580-9.

Nutt JG, Horak FB, Bloem BR. Milestones in gait, balance, and falling. Mov Disord . 2011;26(6):1166-74.

Opara J, Mehlich K, Bielecki A. Walking index for spinal cord injury. Ortop Traumatol Rehabil. 2007;9(2):122-7.

Orr R, Raymond J, Fiatarone Singh M. Efficacy of progressive resistance training on balance performance in older adults : a systematic review of randomized controlled trials. Sports Med. 2008;38(4):317-43.

Pascual-Leone A, Valls-Sole J, Wassermann EM, Brasil-Neto J, Cohen LG, Hallett M. Effects of focal transcranial magnetic stimulation on simple reaction time to acoustic, visual and somatosensory stimuli. Brain. 1992;115 (Pt 4):1045-59.

Patla A, Frank JS, Winter DA, Rietdyk S, Prentice SD, Prasad S. Age-related changes in balance control system: initiation of stepping. Clin Biomech. 1993;8:179-84.

Peters B. Driving performance and workload assessment of drivers with tetraplegia: an adaptation evaluation framework. J Rehabil Res Dev. 2001;38(2):215-24.

Petersen NT, Pyndt HS, Nielsen JB. Investigating human motor control by transcranial magnetic stimulation. Exp Brain Res. 2003;152(1):1-16.

Peterson EW, Cho CC, von Koch L, Finlayson ML. Injurious falls among middle aged and older adults with multiple sclerosis. Arch Phys Med Rehabil. 2008;89(6):1031-7.

Planton M, Peiffer S, Albucher JF, Barbeau EJ, Tardy J, Pastor J, et al. Neuropsychological outcome after a first symptomatic ischaemic stroke with 'good recovery'. Eur J Neurol. 2011. DOI: 10.1111/j.1468-1331.2011.03450.x (Epub ahead of print, June 1.).

Platz T, van Kaick S, Moller L, Freund S, Winter T, Kim IH. Impairment-oriented training and adaptive motor cortex reorganisation after stroke: a fTMS study. J Neurol. 2005;252(11):1363-71.

Poppele R, Bosco G. Sophisticated spinal contributions to motor control. Trends Neurosci. 2003;26(5):269-76.

Post MW, Van Lieshout G, Seelen HA, Snoek GJ, Ijzerman MJ, Pons C. Measurement properties of the short version of the Van Lieshout test for arm/hand function of persons with tetraplegia after spinal cord injury. Spinal Cord. 2006;44(12):763-71.

Raineteau O, Schwab ME. Plasticity of motor systems after incomplete spinal cord injury. Nat Rev Neurosci. 2001;2(4):263-73.

Ramón y Cajal S. Degeneration and Regeneration of the Nervous System. Oxford University Press; New York, NY, USA. 1928.

Richards CL, Olney SJ. Hemiparetic gait following stroke. Part II: Recovery and physical therapy. Gait Posture. 1996;4(2):149-62.

Richards JS, Meredith RL, Nepomuceno C, Fine PR, Bennett G. Psycho-social aspects of chronic pain in spinal cord injury. Pain. 1980;8(3):355-66.

Riener R, Lunenburger L, Maier IC, Colombo G, Dietz V. Locomotor Training in Subjects with Sensori-Motor Deficits: An Overview of the Robotic Gait Orthosis Lokomat. J Healthcare Eng. 2010;1:197-216.

Rintala DH, Loubser PG, Castro J, Hart KA, Fuhrer MJ. Chronic pain in a community-based sample of men with spinal cord injury: prevalence, severity, and relationship with impairment, disability, handicap, and subjective well-being. Arch Phys Med Rehabil. 1998;79(6):604-14.

Rogers ME, Rogers NL, Takeshima N, Islam MM. Methods to assess and improve the physical parameters associated with fall risk in older adults. Prev Med. 2003;36(3):255-64.

Rosnow RL, Rosenthal R. Computing Contrasts, Effect Sizes, and Counternulls on Other People's Published Data: General Procedures for Research Consumers. Psychol Methods. 1996;1(4):331-40.

Rossier P, Wade DT. Validity and reliability comparison of 4 mobility measures in patients presenting with neurologic impairment. Arch Phys Med Rehabil. 2001;82(1):9-13.

Rudhe C, van Hedel HJ. Upper extremity function in persons with tetraplegia: relationships between strength, capacity, and the spinal cord independence measure. Neurorehabil Neural Repair. 2009;23(5):413-21.

Ruger HA, B. S. On the growth curve of certain characters in man (males). Ann Eugenic. 1927;2:76-110.

Sabatier MJ, Redmon N, Schwartz G, English AW. Treadmill training promotes axon regeneration in injured peripheral nerves. Exp Neurol. 2008;211(2):489-93.

Salaffi F, Stancati A, Silvestri CA, Ciapetti A, Grassi W. Minimal clinically important changes in chronic musculoskeletal pain intensity measured on a numerical rating scale. Eur J Pain. 2004;8(4):283-91.

Schuck P, Zwingmann C. The 'smallest real difference' as a measure of sensitivity to change: a critical analysis. Int J Rehabil Res. 2003;26(2):85-91.

Schunemann HJ, Jaeschke R, Cook DJ, Bria WF, El-Solh AA, Ernst A, et al. An official ATS statement: grading the quality of evidence and strength of recommendations in ATS guidelines and recommendations. Am J Resp Crit Care. 2006;174(5):605-14.

Schwartz S, Cohen ME, Herbison GJ, Shah A. Relationship between two measures of upper extremity strength: manual muscle test compared to hand-held myometry. Arch Phys Med Rehabil. 1992;73(11):1063-8.

Scivoletto G, Di Donna V. Prediction of walking recovery after spinal cord injury. Brain Res Bull. 2009;78(1):43-51.

Scivoletto G, Morganti B, Molinari M. Early versus delayed inpatient spinal cord injury rehabilitation: an Italian study. Arch Phys Med Rehabil. 2005;86(3):512-6.

Scivoletto G, Morganti B, Cosentino E, Molinari M. Utility of delayed spinal cord injury rehabilitation: an Italian study. Neurol Sci. 2006;27(2):86-90.

Scivoletto G, Romanelli A, Mariotti A, Marinucci D, Tamburella F, Mammone A, et al. Clinical factors that affect walking level and performance in chronic spinal cord lesion patients. Spine. 2008;33(3):259-64.

Sekhon LH, Fehlings MG. Epidemiology, demographics, and pathophysiology of acute spinal cord injury. Spine. 2001;26(24 Suppl):S2-12.

Semerjian TZ, Montague SM, Dominguez JF, Davidian AM, de Leon RD. Enhancement of quality of life and body satisfaction through the use of adapted exercise devices for individuals with spinal cord injuries. Top Spinal Cord Inj Rehabil. 2005;11(2):95-108.

Shah PK, Stevens JE, Gregory CM, Pathare NC, Jayaraman A, Bickel SC, et al. Lower-extremity muscle cross-sectional area after incomplete spinal cord injury. Arch Phys Med Rehabil. 2006;87(6):772-8.

Shields RK. Muscular, skeletal, and neural adaptations following spinal cord injury. J Orthop Sports Phys Ther. 2002;32(2):65-74.

Shumway-Cook A, Horak FB. Assessing the influence of sensory interaction of balance. Suggestion from the field. Phys Ther. 1986;66(10):1548-50.

Shumway-Cook A, Woollacott MH. Motor Control: Theory and practical applications (2nd edition). Lippincott Williams and Wilkins; Baltimore, MD, USA. 2001.

Siddall PJ. Management of neuropathic pain following spinal cord injury: now and in the future. Spinal Cord. 2009;47(5):352-9.

Siddall PJ, Taylor DA, Cousins MJ. Classification of pain following spinal cord injury. Spinal Cord. 1997;35(2):69-75.

Siddall PJ, McClelland JM, Rutkowski SB, Cousins MJ. A longitudinal study of the prevalence and characteristics of pain in the first 5 years following spinal cord injury. Pain. 2003;103(3):249-57.

Sipski ML, Jackson AB, Gomez-Marin O, Estores I, Stein A. Effects of gender on neurologic and functional recovery after spinal cord injury. Arch Phys Med Rehabil. 2004;85(11):1826-36.

Sisto SA, Dyson-Hudson T. Dynamometry testing in spinal cord injury. J Rehabil Res Dev. 2007;44(1):123-36.

Skinner RD, Houle JD, Reese NB, Berry CL, Garcia-Rill E. Effects of exercise and fetal spinal cord implants on the H-reflex in chronically spinalized adult rats. Brain Res. 1996;729(1):127-31.

Sollerman C, Ejeskar A. Sollerman hand function test. A standardised method and its use in tetraplegic patients. Scand J Plast Recons. 1995;29(2):167-76.

Solomon AC, Stout JC, Weaver M, Queller S, Tomusk A, Whitlock KB, et al. Ten-year rate of longitudinal change in neurocognitive and motor function in prediagnosis Huntington disease. Mov Disord. 2008;23(13):1830-6.

Spiess MR, Muller RM, Rupp R, Schuld C, van Hedel HJ. Conversion in ASIA impairment scale during the first year after traumatic spinal cord injury. J Neurotrauma. 2009;26(11):2027-36.

Spirduso WW. Reaction and movement time as a function of age and physical activity level. J Gerontol. 1975;30(4):435-40.

Spooren AI, Janssen-Potten YJ, Snoek GJ, Ijzerman MJ, Kerckhofs E, Seelen HA. Rehabilitation outcome of upper extremity skilled performance in persons with cervical spinal cord injuries. J Rehabil Med. 2008;40(8):637-44.

Steeves JD, Lammertse D, Curt A, Fawcett JW, Tuszynski MH, Ditunno JF, et al. Guidelines for the conduct of clinical trials for spinal cord injury (SCI) as developed by the ICCP panel: clinical trial outcome measures. Spinal Cord. 2007;45(3):206-21.

Sullivan KJ, Brown DA, Klassen T, Mulroy S, Ge T, Azen SP, et al. Effects of task-specific locomotor and strength training in adults who were ambulatory after stroke: results of the STEPS randomized clinical trial. Phys Ther. 2007;87(12):1580-602; discussion 603-7.

Sumida M, Fujimoto M, Tokuhiro A, Tominaga T, Magara A, Uchida R. Early rehabilitation effect for traumatic spinal cord injury. Arch Phys Med Rehabil. 2001;82(3):391-5.

Taricco M, Apolone G, Colombo C, Filardo G, Telaro E, Liberati A. Functional status in patients with spinal cord injury: a new standardized measurement scale. Gruppo Interdisciplinare Valutazione Interventi Riabilitativi. Arch Phys Med Rehabil. 2000;81(9):1173-80.

Teixeira-Salmela LF, Nadeau S, McBride I, Olney SJ. Effects of muscle strengthening and physical conditioning training on temporal, kinematic and kinetic variables during gait in chronic stroke survivors. J Rehabil Med. 2001;33(2):53-60.

Thomas SL, Gorassini MA. Increases in corticospinal tract function by treadmill training after incomplete spinal cord injury. J Neurophysiol. 2005;94(4):2844-55.

Tooth L, McKenna K, Geraghty T. Rehabilitation outcomes in traumatic spinal cord injury in Australia: functional status, length of stay and discharge setting. Spinal Cord. 2003;41(4):220-30.

Trimble MH, Kukulka CG, Behrman AL. The effect of treadmill gait training on low-frequency depression of the soleus H-reflex: comparison of a spinal cord injured man to normal subjects. Neurosci Lett. 1998;246(3):186-8.

Tseng GF, Prince DA. Structural and functional alterations in rat corticospinal neurons after axotomy. J Neurophysiol. 1996;75(1):248-67.

Vallery H, Duschau-Wicke A, Riener R. Generaliued elasticities improve patient-cooperative control of rehabilitation robots. In IEEE Int Conf on Rehabilitation Robotics (ICORR). 2009a:535-41.

Vallery H, Duschau-Wicke A, Riener R. Optimized passive dynamics improve transparency of haptic devices. In IEEE Int Conf Robot Aut (ICRA). 2009b:301-6.

van den Bogert AJ, Pavol MJ, Grabiner MD. Response time is more important than walking speed for the ability of older adults to avoid a fall after a trip. J Biomech. 2002;35(2):199-205.

van Hedel HJ. Gait speed in relation to categories of functional ambulation after spinal cord injury. Neurorehabil Neural Repair. 2009;23(4):343-50.

van Hedel HJ, Dietz V. Walking during daily life can be validly and responsively assessed in subjects with a spinal cord injury. Neurorehabil Neural Repair. 2009;23(2):117-24.

van Hedel HJ, Dietz V. Rehabilitation of locomotion after spinal cord injury. Restor Neurol Neurosci. 2010;28(1):123-34.

van Hedel HJ, Wirth B, Dietz V. Limits of locomotor ability in subjects with a spinal cord injury. Spinal Cord. 2005a;43(10):593-603.

van Hedel HJ, Wirz M, Dietz V. Assessing walking ability in subjects with spinal cord injury: validity and reliability of 3 walking tests. Arch Phys Med Rehabil. 2005b;86(2):190-6.

van Hedel HJ, Wirz M, Curt A. Improving walking assessment in subjects with an incomplete spinal cord injury: responsiveness. Spinal Cord. 2006;44(6):352-6.

van Hedel HJ, Dietz V, Curt A. Assessment of walking speed and distance in subjects with an incomplete spinal cord injury. Neurorehabil Neural Repair. 2007a;21(4):295-301.

van Hedel HJ, Murer C, Dietz V, Curt A. The amplitude of lower leg motor evoked potentials is a reliable measure when controlled for torque and motor task. J Neurol. 2007b;254(8):1089-98.

van Hedel HJ, Wirz M, Dietz V. Standardized assessment of walking capacity after spinal cord injury: the European network approach. Neurol Res. 2008;30(1):61-73.

van Hedel HJ, Wirth B, Curt A. Ankle motor skill is intact in spinal cord injury, unlike stroke: implications for rehabilitation. Neurology. 2010;74(16):1271-8.

van Hedel HJ, Dokladal P, Hotz-Boendermaker S. Mismatch Between Investigator-Determined and Patient-Reported Independence After Spinal Cord Injury: Consequences for Rehabilitation and Trials. Neurorehabil Neural Repair. 2011. DOI: 10.1177/1545968311407518 (Epub ahead of print, June 2.).

van Middendorp JJ, Hosman AJ, Pouw MH, Van de Meent H. ASIA impairment scale conversion in traumatic SCI: is it related with the ability to walk? A descriptive comparison with functional ambulation outcome measures in 273 patients. Spinal Cord. 2009;47(7):555-60.

van Middendorp JJ, Hosman AJ, Donders AR, Pouw MH, Ditunno JF, Curt A, et al. A clinical prediction rule for ambulation outcomes after traumatic spinal cord injury: a longitudinal cohort study. Lancet. 2011;377(9770):1004-10.

van Tuijl JH, Janssen-Potten YJ, Seelen HA. Evaluation of upper extremity motor function tests in tetraplegics. Spinal Cord. 2002;40(2):51-64.

Visintin M, Barbeau H. The effects of body weight support on the locomotor pattern of spastic paretic patients. Can J Neurol Sci. 1989;16(3):315-25.

Waters RL, Adkins RH, Yakura JS, Sie I. Motor and sensory recovery following incomplete paraplegia. Arch Phys Med Rehabil. 1994a;75(1):67-72.

Waters RL, Adkins RH, Yakura JS, Sie I. Motor and sensory recovery following incomplete tetraplegia. Arch Phys Med Rehabil. 1994b;75(3):306-11.

Weiss A, Suzuki T, Bean J, Fielding RA. High intensity strength training improves strength and functional performance after stroke. Am J Phys Med Rehabil. 2000;79(4):369-76.

Welford AT. Motor Performance. In: Birren JE, Schaie KW, editors. Handbook of the psychology of aging. Van Nostrand Reinhold Co; New York, NY, USA. 1977.

Wickelgren WA. Speed-accuracy tradeoff and information processing dynamics. Acta Psychol. 1977;41:67-85.

Winchester P, McColl R, Querry R, Foreman N, Mosby J, Tansey K, et al. Changes in supraspinal activation patterns following robotic locomotor therapy in motor-incomplete spinal cord injury. Neurorehabil Neural Repair. 2005;19(4):313-24.

Wirth B, van Hedel HJ, Curt A. Ankle paresis in incomplete spinal cord injury: relation to corticospinal conductivity and ambulatory capacity. J Clin Neurophysiol. 2008a;25(4):210-7.

Wirth B, van Hedel HJ, Kometer B, Dietz V, Curt A. Changes in activity after a complete spinal cord injury as measured by the Spinal Cord Independence Measure II (SCIM II). Neurorehabil Neural Repair. 2008b;22(3):279-87.

Wirth B, van Hedel HJ, Curt A. Ankle dexterity remains intact in patients with incomplete spinal cord injury in contrast to stroke patients. Exp Brain Res. 2008c;191(3):353-61.

Wirz M, Muller R, Bastiaenen C. Falls in persons with spinal cord injury: validity and reliability of the Berg Balance Scale. Neurorehabil Neural Repair. 2009;24(1):70-7.

Wirz M, van Hedel HJ, Rupp R, Curt A, Dietz V. Muscle force and gait performance: relationships after spinal cord injury. Arch Phys Med Rehabil. 2006;87(9):1218-22.

Wirz M, Zemon DH, Rupp R, Scheel A, Colombo G, Dietz V, et al. Effectiveness of automated locomotor training in patients with chronic incomplete spinal cord injury: a multicenter trial. Arch Phys Med Rehabil. 2005;86(4):672-80.

Woolley SM, Czaja SJ, Drury CG. An assessment of falls in elderly men and women. J Gerontol A Biol Sci Med Sci. 1997;52(2):M80-7.

Wrigley PJ, Gustin SM, Macey PM, Nash PG, Gandevia SC, Macefield VG, Siddall PJ, Henderson LA. Anatomical changes in human motor cortex and motor pathways following complete thoracic spinal cord injury. Cereb Cortex. 2009;19(1):224-32.

Wyndaele M, Wyndaele JJ. Incidence, prevalence and epidemiology of spinal cord injury: what learns a worldwide literature survey? Spinal Cord. 2006;44(9):523-9.

Yang JF, Norton J, Nevett-Duchcherer J, Roy FD, Gross DP, Gorassini MA. Volitional muscle strength in the legs predicts changes in walking speed following locomotor training in people with chronic spinal cord injury. Phys Ther. 2011;91(6):931-43.

Yang JF, Stein RB, Jhamandas J, Gordon T. Motor unit numbers and contractile properties after spinal cord injury. Ann Neurol. 1990;28(4):496-502.

Yardley L, Beyer N, Hauer K, Kempen G, Piot-Ziegler C, Todd C. Development and initial validation of the Falls Efficacy Scale-International (FES-I). Age Ageing. 2005;34(6):614-9.

Yavuz N, Tezyurek M, Akyuz M. A comparison of two functional tests in quadriplegia: the quadriplegia index of function and the functional independence measure. Spinal Cord. 1998;36(12):832-7.

11 Abbreviations

4FTRWS	Four functional tasks relevant to wheelchair seating
5-AML	Five additional mobility and locomotor items
6MAT	Six Minutes Arm Test
6MWT	Six Minutes Walk Test
8MW	Eight Meter Walk Test
10MWT	Ten Meter Walk Test
50FWT	Fifty Foot Walk Test
ADL	Activities of daily living
AIS	ASIA Impairment Scale
AMS	ASIA motor score
ASIA	American Spinal Injury Association
AWAnT	Arm Wingate Anaerobic Testing
BBS	Berg Balance Scale
BI	Barthel Index
CRT	Choice response time
CUE	Capabilities of Upper Extremity
DPR	Delayed Plantar Response
EMG	Electromyography
FES-I	Falls Efficacy Scale, international version
FIM	Functional Independence Measure
FIM-L	Functional Independence Measure – Locomotion
FRT	Functional Reach Test
GRASSP	Graded and Redefined Assessment of Strength, Sensibility and Prehension

11. Abbreviations

GRT	Grasp and Release Test
ICC	Intraclass correlation coefficient
iSCI	Incomplete spinal cord injury
ISTT	Independent Samples T Test
KBS	Klein-Bell ADL Scale
LED	Light emitting diode
LEMS	Lower extremity motor score
MAIDS	Mobility Aids
MCAP	Motor amplitudes of the compound action potentials
MCS	Motor Capacity Scale
MBI	Modified Barthel Index
MEP	Motor evoked potentials
MMS	Mini Mental Status Examination Test
MMT	Manual muscle testing
MRR	Motor recovery rate
MWUT	Mann-Whitney U Test
NCV	Nerve conduction velocity
PCI	Physical Cost Index
Prosp.	Prospective
QIF	Quadriplegia Index of Function
RAGT	Robot-assisted gait training
Retrosp.	Retrospective
RCT	Randomized controlled trial
RET	Reaction and Execution Test
SCI	Spinal cord injury
SCI-ARMI	Spinal Cord Injury Ability Realization Measurement Index

11. Abbreviations

SCIM	Spinal Cord Independence Measure
SEP	Somatosensory evoked potentials
SHFT	Sollerman Hand Function Test
SRD	Smallest real difference
ST	Strength training
TA	Tibialis anterior
THAQ	Tetraplegia Hand Activity Questionnaire
TMS	Transcranial magnetic stimulation
TUG	Timed Up and Go
UEMS	Upper extremity motor score
VFM	Valutazione Funzionale Mielolesi
VLT	Van Lieshout Test
VLT-SV	Van Lieshout Test – Short Version
VRI	Voluntary Response Index
WISCI	Walking Index for Spinal Cord Injury
WST	Wheelchair Skills Test

12 Curriculum vitae

Name | Rob Labruyère
Date of Birth | 28th of August 1980
Citizen of | Davos, Switzerland and Rotterdam, the Netherlands

Education
2008 – 2011 | PhD at ETH Zurich, Switzerland
Research conducted at the Spinal Cord Injury Centre, University Hospital Balgrist, Zurich
2002 – 2007 | Master of Science in Human Movement Sciences and Sport at ETH Zurich, Switzerland
2000 – 2002 | Studies of Biology at University of Zurich, Switzerland
1993 – 2000 | High School, Schweizerische Alpine Mittelschule Davos, Switzerland

Working Experience
2011 | Medical Technical Assistant (10%), Prodorso - Center for Spine Medicine, Zurich
2008 - 2011 | Medical Technical Assistant (10%), Neurophysiology Department, University Hospital Balgrist, Zurich

Oral Presentations
R. Labruyère, A. Agarwala, A. Curt; "Ideal Timing and Outcome

Instruments for Rehabilitation of the Spinal Cord Injured Patient - A Systematic Review", Editorial Board Meeting "Spine", Chicago, USA, May 2010.

Poster Presentations

R. Labruyère, H. van Hedel; "Is automated locomotor training better than strength training after incomplete spinal cord injury?". 13th annual ZNZ Symposium, Zurich, Switzerland, Sept. 2010.

R. Labruyère, H. van Hedel; "Is automated locomotor training better than strength training after incomplete spinal cord injury?". 18th Congress of the International Society of Electrophysiology and Kinesiology, Aalborg, Denmark, June 2010.

R. Labruyère, M. Wirz, H. van Hedel; "Response time of the lower extremity in people with incomplete spinal cord injury - a feasibility study". 48th ISCoS Annual Scientific Meeting, Florence, Italy, October 2009.

R. Labruyère, M. Wirz, H. van Hedel; "Response time of the lower extremity in people with incomplete spinal cord injury - a feasibility study". 12th annual ZNZ Symposium, Zurich, Switzerland, Sept. 2009.

R. Labruyère, H. van Hedel; "Specific locomotor versus unspecific weight training and their effects on corticospinal conductivity and other outcomes in subjects with chronic incomplete spinal cord injury". Spinal Research Network Meeting, London, UK, Aug. 2008.

Awards

The **Fürst Donnersmarck Stiftung** (Berlin, Germany) commended this work for exceptional scientific achievements in the field of rehabilitation.

13 Publications

Labruyère R, Agarwala A, Curt A. Rehabilitation in spine and spinal cord trauma. Spine. 2010;35(21 Suppl):S259-62.

Labruyère R, van Hedel H. Instrument validity and reliability of a choice response time test for incomplete spinal cord injured subjects: relationship with function. Arch Phys Med Rehabil. 2011;92(9):1443-9.

Labruyère R, van Hedel H. Curve Walking Is Not Better Than Straight Walking in Estimating Ambulation-Related Domains After Incomplete Spinal Cord Injury. Arch Phys Med Rehabil. 2012;93(5):796-801.

Labruyère R, van Hedel H. Slowed Down: Response Time Deficits in Well- Recovered Subjects With Incomplete Spinal Cord Injury. Arch Phys Med Rehabil. 2013;94:2020-6.

Labruyère R, van Hedel H. Strength training versus robot-assisted gait training after incomplete spinal cord injury: a randomized pilot study in patients depending on walking assistance. J Neuroeng Rehabil 2014;9;11(1):4

14 Acknowledgement

PD Dr. Hubertus Johannes Antonius van Hedel, who made this thesis possible by believing in me and scraping together the funding. It was exceedingly pleasant working with him and I profited a lot. He also allowed me to express my Dutch roots and to make fun of his German, I owe him big time!

Prof. Urs Boutellier, for agreeing to be the head of my committee and giving me the chance to do my PhD thesis outside the ETH Zurich at the University Hospital Balgrist. His inputs were very precious.

Prof. Robert Riener, for being the co-referee of my thesis and for his valuable questions at our meetings. Sorry that the Lokomat flopped in chapters 6 and 7.

Prof. Armin Curt, for letting me fiddle around with my thesis in his lab and for giving me the opportunity to write the review, Dr. Martin Schubert and Dr. Gertraut Lindemann for letting me stick needles into living objects, and Dr. Marc Bolliger, for taking care of Armin's lab and for exchanging the latest Mac infos.

All PhD students at the Paralab for the funny and profitable ambiance they created, and especially Michèle Hubli, Sandra Keller and Chuck Norris who contributed to a very comfortable atmosphere in our room.

Marion Zimmerli, for being such a nice and productive student.

All other colleagues at Paralab, it was a great place to work.

14. Acknowledgement

All who participated as subjects in my studies, especially P01, P02, P03, P04, P05, P06, P07, P08 and P09 for your endurance and patience!

Thierry "the bird" Perriard, for designing and Lino Cutting the wonderful cover!

My family, for always being there for me. Mam, please don't show this thesis to people who are not interested! Dad, please tell her again! Menno, blijf kuieren!

Corinne, I owe you everything, you're awesome and gorgeous!!

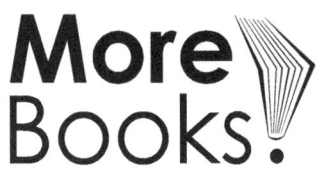

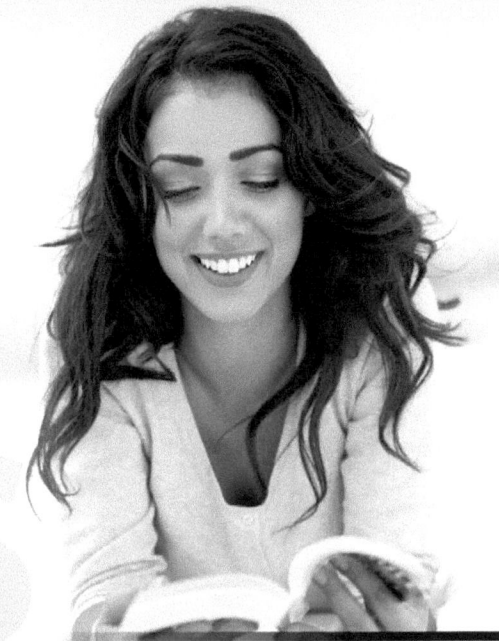

i want morebooks!

Buy your books fast and straightforward online - at one of world's fastest growing online book stores! Environmentally sound due to Print-on-Demand technologies.

Buy your books online at
www.get-morebooks.com

Kaufen Sie Ihre Bücher schnell und unkompliziert online – auf einer der am schnellsten wachsenden Buchhandelsplattformen weltweit! Dank Print-On-Demand umwelt- und ressourcenschonend produziert.

Bücher schneller online kaufen
www.morebooks.de

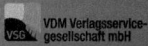

VDM Verlagsservicegesellschaft mbH
Heinrich-Böcking-Str. 6-8   Telefon: +49 681 3720 174   info@vdm-vsg.de
D - 66121 Saarbrücken   Telefax: +49 681 3720 1749 www.vdm-vsg.de

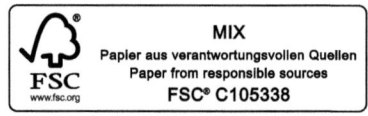

Printed by Books on Demand GmbH, Norderstedt / Germany